W9-ANX-290

Bountiful Health,
Boundless Energy,
Brilliant Youth
The Facts About DHEA

Dr. Neecie Moore

Charis Publishing Co., Inc.

A Charis Publishing Book

Published by Charis Publishing Co., Inc.
11551 Forest Central Drive
PO Box 740607
Dallas, Texas, 75243

Cover by Mat Hames and David Colister
Photo by Mickey Torres

All Rights Reserved. No part of this book may be reproduced in any form without written permission from Charis Publishing Co., Inc. This book is intended to be a reference only. It is not to be used for diagnosis for the treatment of disease. Before making changes in your diet, your medication or your exercise program, consult with your physician. In stories and examples, all names have been changed, although all stories are used with permission.

Copyright © 1994 by Charis Publishing Co., Inc.

Printed in the United States of America.

Library of Congress Catalog Card Number: 94-850941

Dr. Neecie Moore
Bountiful Health, Boundless Energy, Brilliant Youth:
The Facts about DHEA
First Edition
$12.95 Softcover

To my dear friends,
Sam
and
Bill

In loving memory of:
Mamaw
and
Aunt Mamie

TABLE OF CONTENTS

INTRODUCTION – WHAT IS DEHYDROEPIANDROSTERONE? 11
    DHEA IS PRODUCED IN OUR BODIES
    THE FDA RULES ON DHEA
    THE IMPORTANCE OF FORMULATING NATURAL PRODUCTS
        FROM THE WILD MEXICAN YAM

CHAPTER ONE – THE MIRACLE IN THE MEXICAN YAM 15

CHAPTER TWO – DHEA: ANTIOBESITY AGENT; DHEA AND
                FAT LOSS 18
    WHY WEIGHT MAINTENANCE IS IMPORTANT
    WHY MANY AMERICANS ARE OVERWEIGHT
    CAUSES OF OBESITY
    DHEA AND OBESITY: STUDIES IN ANIMALS
    FOOD DEPRIVATION NOT NECESSARY
        WITH DHEA TREATMENT
    DHEA BLOCKS THE PRODUCTION OF FAT
    DHEA ACCELERATES WEIGHT LOSS
    DHEA CURBS HUNGER
    HOW DHEA WORKS AS AN ANTIOBESITY AGENT
    "ROCKIN' ROBBIN" NEVER FELT (OR LOOKED) BETTER!

CHAPTER THREE – DIABETES AND DHEA 32
    TYPE I AND TYPE II DIABETES
    INSULIN: ONCE THOUGHT A "CURE ALL"
    DIABETES: THE THIRD LEADING CAUSE OF DEATH
    THE IMPORTANCE OF PREVENTION
    THE SYMPTOMS AND CAUSES OF DIABETES
    BEING CAUTIOUS AND SELF TREATMENT
    DHEA AS AN ANTIDIABETES AGENT
    A SUCCESS STORY FROM A PHYSICIAN

CHAPTER FOUR – THE CARDIOVASCULAR SYSTEM AND
              THE POWERFUL EFFECTS OF DHEA 38
    THE PREVALENCE OF CORONARY DISEASE
    OUR HEART'S GREATEST ENEMY: ATHEROSCLEROSIS
    CARDIOVASCULAR HEALTH
    DHEA LEVELS AND HEART DISEASE
    SEX-RELATED DIFFERENCES
    DIFFERENCES IN DHEA LEVELS IN DIFFERENT RACES
        AGE, CARDIOVASCULAR DISEASE, AND DHEA LEVELS

CARDIOVASCULAR RISK AND DHEA
SMOKING, CARDIOVASCULAR DISEASE AND DHEA
STRESS AND DHEA
TYPE A BEHAVIOR AND DHEA
DHEA AND ATHEROSCLEROSIS
VARIOUS STUDIES ABOUT CARDIOVASCULAR DISEASE
    AND DHEA
ADMINISTERING DHEA TO CARDIOVASCULAR PATIENTS
CONCLUSIONS ABOUT DHEA AND CARDIOVASCULAR
    DISEASE
A "HEART-FELT" STORY

CHAPTER FIVE – MENOPAUSE, HORMONE REPLACEMENT THERAPY,
             AND OSTEOPOROSIS: DHEA TO THE RESCUE 54
WHAT IS MENOPAUSE?
THE SYMPTOMS OF MENOPAUSE
ONCE UPON A TIME ELDERLY WOMEN WERE HONORED
HOT FLASHES AND FLUSHES
SWELLING AND BLOATING
VAGINAL DRYNESS
ADDRESSING MENOPAUSE AND HORMONAL IMBALANCES
    WITH MOTHER NATURES' TREATMENTS
HORMONAL PRODUCTION THROUGH MENOPAUSE
STRENGTHENING AND NOURISHING YOUR ADRENAL SYSTEM
HORMONAL REPLACEMENT: PROS AND CONS
HORMONAL REPLACEMENT: SYNTHETIC OR NATURAL?
WHY PHYSICIANS PRESCRIBE SYNTHETIC HORMONES
OSTEOPOROSIS
WHEN DOES OSTEOPOROSIS OCCUR?
ABOUT OUR BONES AND OSTEOPOROSIS
THE RISK OF FRACTURES
THE MOST POWERFUL PREVENTION: EXERCISE
ANOTHER GREAT PREVENTION: SEXUAL ACTIVITY
OTHER NATURAL TREATMENTS FOR OSTEOPOROSIS
NATURAL PROGESTERONE CAN REVERSE OSTEOPOROSIS
WHY NATURAL PROGESTERONE IS SO EFFECTIVE
THE GOOD NEWS

CHAPTER SIX – PREMENSTRUAL SYNDROME: THE BATTLE OF THE
             HORMONES AND THE EFFECTS OF DHEA 71
THE AWFUL SYMPTOMS OF PMS
THE CAUSES OF PMS
THE BATTLE OF THE HORMONES

THE NORMAL RISE AND FALL OF HORMONES
HAVING YOUR HORMONES CHECKED
TREATING PMS: PRESCRIPTION DRUGS OR NATURAL PRODUCTS
EXERCISE AND PMS
OTHER PRACTICAL REMEDIES
PSYCHOTHERAPY AND PMS
NATURAL PROGESTERONE AND PMS
"IT'S LIKE A MIRACLE"

CHAPTER SEVEN – DHEA: CAN IT LOWER CHOLESTEROL? 85
CHOLESTEROL ≠ FAT
THE GOOD GUYS AND THE BAD GUYS OF CHOLESTEROL
IDEALS LEVELS OF HDL AND LDL
SYMPTOM OF HIGH LDL AND LOW HDL CHOLESTEROL
NATURAL TREATMENTS FOR HIGH CHOLESTEROL
NATURAL TREATMENT TO LOWER HDL LEVELS
RESEARCH ABOUT DHEA AND CHOLESTEROL
ONE WOMAN'S SUCCESS STORY

CHAPTER EIGHT – DHEA'S EFFECT ON ARTHRITIS AND MULTIPLE ..
                    SCLEROSIS 92
ARTHRITIS
DHEA TREATMENT OF ARTHRITIS
MULTIPLE SCLEROSIS
USE OF DHEA IN TREATING MULTIPLE SCLEROSIS

CHAPTER NINE – DHEA: AN ANTIDEPRESSANT? 96
WHO IS DEPRESSED?
SYMPTOMS OF DEPRESSION
WHAT CAUSES DEPRESSION
HOW TO HELP WHEN SOMEONE YOU KNOW IS DEPRESSED
TREATING DEPRESSION
TREATING DEPRESSION NATURALLY
RESEARCH ABOUT DHEA AND DEPRESSION
WHAT DOCTORS SAY ABOUT DHEA AND DEPRESSION
COUPLE FINDS RELIEF FROM DEPRESSION

CHAPTER TEN – DHEA AND THE LIVER: THE HOUSE OF
                    THE SOUL 108
THE MANY FUNCTIONS OF THE LIVER
THE LIVER PROVIDES THE BUILDING BLOCKS (PRECURSORS)
        FOR HORMONES
DETOXIFICATION: THE MAJOR JOB OF THE LIVER
DHEA AND THE LIVER

CHAPTER ELEVEN – THE DEVASTATIONS OF CANCER, THE
                        PROMISE OF DHEA TREATMENTS 114
    THE TRAGEDIES OF CANCER
    TOXIC TREATMENT FOR CANCER PREVAILS
    DHEA AND CANCER PREVENTION
    BREAST CANCER
    DHEA AND BREAST CANCER
    CANCER, SEX HORMONES, AND DHEA
    GYNECOLOGIC CANCERS
    DHEA'S EFFECT ON CANCER IN ANIMAL STUDIES

CHAPTER TWELVE – AGING, MEMORY AND ALZHEIMER'S
                        DISEASE: HOW DHEA CAN HELP 122
    THE FOUNTAIN OF YOUTH
    THE SEARCH FOR LONGEVITY GOES ON AND ON . . .
    HOW LONG CAN WE LIVE?
    ABOUT OUR WONDERFUL SENIOR CITIZENS
    CAUSES OF PREMATURE AGING
    NATURAL TREATMENTS FOR PREMATURE AGING
    USING MEDITATION TO STAY YOUNG
    DHEA: YOU CAN STAY YOUNG!
    ALZHEIMER'S DISEASE
    CAUSES OF ALZHEIMER'S DISEASE
    NATURAL TREATMENT OF ALZHEIMER'S DISEASE
    A HEART BREAKING STORY TO LEARN FROM

CHAPTER THIRTEEN – DHEA: HOPE FOR AIDS PATIENTS? 135
    CAUSE OF AIDS
    VAST NUMBERS OF CASES REPORTED
    ASTOUNDING NUMBERS OF DEATHS
    AIDS AFFECTS BOTH MEN AND WOMEN
    SYMPTOMS OF THE DISEASE
    HOW HIV INFECTS THE SYSTEM
    NATURAL TREATMENTS FOR HIV AND AIDS
    FACTS ABOUT AIDS
    PREVENTION OF AIDS
    AIDS PATIENTS TAKE CHARGE
    RESEARCH ABOUT DHEA WITH AIDS PATIENTS
    NEW HOPE FOR AIDS PATIENTS

CHAPTER FOURTEEN – THE MOST FREQUENTLY ASKED QUESTIONS
                        ABOUT DHEA 148

APPENDIX A – THE BIOCHEMICAL PATHWAY.......................................169

APPENDIX B – THE BIOCHEMISTRY 170

APPENDIX C – WHERE TO GET THE NATURAL
PRECURSOR PRODUCTS 173

SPECIAL NOTE

This book is for reference purposes and is not meant to be nor replace medical advice. The information and material presented is strictly intended for educational purposes. The publishers nor the author are intending to make recommendations about your health care. The purpose of this book is not for self-diagnosis or self-treatment of any illness or disease. Before making changes in your diet, your medication or your exercise program, consult with your physician.

In stories and examples, all names have been changed, although all stories are used with permission.

ACKNOWLEDGEMENTS

I would like to acknowledge all the family members, clients, friends, and colleagues who have cheered me on throughout this project.

Thanks to my friends at High Hopes: Dennis and Alan and the whole group;

Thanks to my friends at the Center for Family Development: Patty, Kimberly, Kay, for covering for me while I was buried;

Thanks to my support group: Ginny, Mary Ellen, Anita, Susan, and Shari, for helping me stay sane and centered;

Thanks to my "brother" Andy and my "sister" Carol, and my "brother" Glen and my "sister" Pat for helping through some difficult days;

Thanks to my pastors, Sidney and Linda Brandon, and my church family in Lavon, Texas who kept me inspired;

Thanks to "Momsy" and Janis for all of the prayers.

Thanks to Gail, Patti, Patty, and Joe for being my friend through it all and always having an encouraging word;

Thanks to my friends, Sam and Linda, Don and Lydia, Bill and Donna, Dick and Nancy, Ray and Diana, Jim and D.J., Lowell and Shirley, Zita, Norma Jean,Bob, John, J.W., Jett, Bridget (my little sis), and the many others who were always cheerleaders for me;

Thanks to Jamie and Kathy for all the support;

Thanks to Missy, Indu, Mickey, Randall, Dale, Dick, Kim, Tempe, Jason, Larry, Steve, Terry, David, Cathy and Rick for all the smiles;

Thanks to Dr. Reg McDaniels for reviewing my manuscript;

Thanks to Dr. Sterling Sightler for saving my mother's life and taking care of her, so she could be here to cheer me on;

Thanks to Dr. Sam Harvey for being a great guide through the dark moments of life;

Thanks to Gary for all the help with the writing, the editing, the proofing; thanks for all your encouragement, support; thanks for believing I could finish this even when I didn't; and thanks for being a trustworthy friend.

and MOST OF ALL thanks to God for strength and courage.

SPECIAL THANKS:

To my mother, "Sissie", who taught me about strength and prayer;
to my dad, "Red", who taught me to work hard;
to my sister, "Ruana", who created the four greatest gifts of my life: Kimberly, Jason,
Paul and Rebekah;
and to my precious girls:
Kelli, Colleen, Andrea,
Jill and Sarah.

INTRODUCTION

===

WHAT IS DEHYDROEPIANDROSTERONE?

Dehydroepiandrosterone . . . Not since Mary Poppin's "supercalifragilisticexpialidocious" has there been such a big word that produced such delightful results. Research has indicated that DHEA has significant anti-obesity, anti-tumor, anti-aging, and anti-cancer effects; that it . . . "may extend your life and make you more youthful while you're alive." (Dean, 1990, p. 95).

After reading just those few words, you might be asking yourself: "So what is this 'stuff'? Where do you get it? And why haven't I ever heard about it before?"

The most amazing answer to that question is that DHEA is produced in our bodies. To fully understand the concept, a short science lesson is in order. If you never enjoyed science in the first place, you might skip this section and move on to Chapter One. For those who are curious and/or want a full scientific understanding of DHEA, let's begin with what it is and how and where it is produced in our bodies.

DHEA IS PRODUCED IN OUR BODIES

Two of the major systems that control our body and its functions are the nervous system and the endocrine system. The nervous system controls the body with the use of nerve impulses, sending messages throughout the body while the endocrine system sends messages more slowly through chemical messengers called hormones. The name hormones was taken from a Greek word, "hormon" which means to "stir up or excite." (Parker, 1993).

These hormones are produced by various glands. The master gland, the pituitary, produces growth hormone and prolactin which control growth and the production of a mother's milk. The thyroid produces thyroxine which controls metabolism, or the way the body uses energy. The parathyroids produce parathormone which regulates calcium levels in the body. The pancreas produces insulin which regulates the body's use of sugar. The testicles produce testosterone which controls the development of the sexual organs and masculine characteristics in males. The ovaries produce oestrogen and progesterone which control the development of sexual organs and feminine characteristics in females. Finally, the adrenal gland produces several hormones, one of which is DHEA.

The adrenal glands are housed in fat just above the kidneys, weighing about five grams each. The right adrenal is pyramid-shaped, while the left one is crescent shaped. Each of them have two major parts, the outer cortex and the central medulla. The cortex produces steroid hormones: aldosterone, cortisol (hydrocortisone), and DHEA. The medulla produces the catecholamines, such as epinephrine and norepinephrine.

DHEA is also produced in the gonads. DHEA is the most abundant hormone in the blood stream (Berdanier et al, 1993). Its concentrations dramatically increase during puberty and then sharply decrease after about age twenty or thirty (Smith et. al, 1975). Perhaps this is one of the reasons that so many refer to it as "the fountain of youth."

THE FDA RULES ON DHEA

Although scientific research validates its many benefits, such as its effectiveness in treating obesity, acting against tumors, cardiovascular disease and some forms of diabetes, it is basically not used in modern medical practice. Research regarding the use and benefits of DHEA treating various maladies is incredibly pervasive. For example, upon entering a program such as MedLine II in the spring of 1994, some 4,533 articles regarding studies involving the use of DHEA are reported. DHEA, because of its decline in the body as one moves into midlife, was produced in synthetic form in the 1940s, 1950s, and 1960s and was available for purchase. Because the FDA views DHEA as experimental, it was taken from the market in 1985, when the FDA issued a press released stating: "FDA has few adverse reaction reports on the drug, but the risks from long-term use are unknown" (Flieger, 1988).

DHEA is very safe (nontoxic), because the body knows how and where to use it for optimum health (Whitaker, 1992). In addition, the body seems to basically ignore the DHEA if it doesn't need it. Some doctors believe that the reason that the FDA withholds its approval on this and other steroid compounds is because so many drug companies are attempting to alter their molecular structure so that they can obtain a patent on the drug (Whitaker, 1992 and Lee, 1993). In addition, Whitaker, (1992) believes the FDA clamps down on substances that are without a patent. Much of the money used to study chemicals is provided by pharmaceutical companies, hoping to get the drug approved and to be granted a patent. Natural substances which are manufactured from whole foods, without an altered molecular substance, are unpatentable, and therefore, unappealing to the pharmaceutical companies.

THE IMPORTANCE OF FORMULATING NATURAL PRODUCTS FROM THE WILD MEXICAN YAM

Many people seem to misunderstand the absence of FDA's approval, and assume it means it is an illegal substance. However, it is NOT illegal, nor dangerous, but has only been tested on a limited basis. Available by prescription only, some physicians remain reluctant to prescribe it and some pharmacies hesitant to stock it. Understanding this dilemma supports the notion of a sense of the miraculous when the Mexican Yam and its benefits were discovered!

1

THE MIRACLE IN THE MEXICAN YAM

The Mexican Yam, *Dioscorea villosa*, was first mentioned for its miraculous uses in 25 B.C. in the Pen Tsao Ching by the Chinese who highly valued the herb (Gladstar, 1993). It was not until this century that there are reports of the Yam being highly sought by pharmaceutical companies. Japanese researchers discovered the value of the Wild Yam in 1936 when they realized that diosgenin was an herbal extract of the yam that was remarkably similar to some of the adrenal hormones (Mowrey, 1986).

An incredible advancement occurred in 1943 when Russel Marker was able to manufacture progesterone from the roots of the Mexican Yam. Some biochemists believe that the biochemical structure of diosgenin is very similar to that of cholesterol, which eventually makes progesterone in the body. Some doctors have proclaimed that diosgenin is not just extremely similar, but that diosgenin "has been made to match natural progesterone exactly" (Kamen, 1993, p. 200).

By the late 1940s and early 1950s, drug companies seeking diosgenin created a booming steroid industry in Mexico. (Bioscience, 1992). They were harvesting the Wild Yam so fast and furiously, and building labs and manufacturing plants,

15

that Mexico's economy experienced some real, temporary benefits. According to a 1951 *Fortune* Magazine article, the steroid industry created "the biggest technological boom ever heard south of the border" (Fortune, 1951).

Perhaps because of its use in the formulation of birth control pills (which are almost a household words among females), the Wild Yam has been "the most widely used herb in the world today" (Gladstar, 1993, p 258).   It provides 50 percent of the raw materials for manufacturing steroids. As a matter of fact, it was the sole source of diosgenin used in birth control pills until alternative plants were discovered recently.   More than two hundred million prescriptions annually are produced and sold where Wild Yam diosgenin is used (Gladstar, 1993).

The miracle of the Wild Yam is best explained by learning about an island so beautifully written about in a 1992 National Geographic article entitled "Under the Spell of the Trobriand Islands." The Trobriand Islands, part of New Guinea, seems to be a magical place, making the title of the article ever so appropriate. The most prized commodity in their culture is the miraculous yam. Every island has a yam house, which is the tallest, and most beautiful structure in the primitive village. The yam is the centerpiece of every social event, being the prized food when there are guests, when there are celebrations, any opportunity which calls for a feast.

However, the yam is not just a tasty dish served in feasts and festivals; it is a sign of wealth and prosperity, symbolizing life and strength. The plants are cared for ever so meticulously, for the major competition between villages, and villagers, is who has grown the longest, most beautiful yam of the season. The harvest time of the yam is the most important event of their year, calling for a month-long festival.

Tending of the yams is done by men, but harvesting is done by village women. Any man who even shows up at a procession of women carrying the yam can be ridiculed or attacked. The punishment, for the serious crime of interrupting such an important procession is to be stripped naked, thrown into the center of the village, and laughed at.

It is also the yam that decides when a boy becomes a man in the Trobriands. When a boy can tend a garden on his own, about age 14 or 15, raising the yam with care, it is time for him to get his own plot of land and his own house.

The yam is a valuable asset, and makes the paramount chief of the village rich. Only the paramount chief is allowed to have many wives, and each wife's family must provide a dowry of sorts, in the form of yam, called a "yam tribute." The real value of the yam is not only in how much a person produces, but in how much a person can give away.

Interestingly enough, these people who develop their lives around the yam, and who feast on yams, are very youthful. They do not know when their birthday is, nor how old they are. They save their celebration for the dancing, the festival, the feast of the yam. In addition, for some unexplained reason, their birthrate is extremely low. Perhaps the yam, their most prized commodity, has provided for them, for many years, the miracles of birth control that steroid drugs and natural hormonal products derived from the Wild Mexican Yam are now being intently sought for in America today.

2

DHEA : AN ANTIOBESITY AGENT
DHEA AND FAT LOSS

The U.S. weight loss industry is a bilion dollar business. Of all the reasons given for this boom, one stands out: "Thin is In!" The thinner the better.

Although there are now "Big and Tall" shops for males and "Plus" or "Woman" shops for females, there is a incredible prejudice regarding overweight people in our country. Overweight people believe they are denied employment and other opportunities simply due to their problems with weight. Cher, in her book, *Forever Fit* (1991), stated: "One recent study revealed that being overweight decreases annual income by an average of $4,000 a year per person. Research has also shown that, fair or not, thin people get promotions and pay raises faster then fat people" (p 38). "Thin is smarter and richer and better paid" (Stuart and Orr, 1987). "Society points its finger in shame at the overweight, making them feel that they are somehow morally weak, that they are gluttons with little strength of character" (Bailey, 1977). All of these quotes illustrate the prejudice we have for overweight people.

Yet, obesity (when the ideal weight for height and bone

structure is exceeded by twenty five percent) and weight remains a major problem. The problem is obvious by the numbers of weight loss clinics, treatment programs for eating disorders, the advertisements for health clubs, and the growth in numbers of support groups such as Overeaters Anonymous. Most overweight people have tried one or more of these programs. However, losing weight is not the main problem for overweight people. Most have lost incredible numbers of pounds on various diets and schemes, only to gain those pounds back, plus more. The main problem is not in losing the weight, but in gaining the weight back. Dr. Kelly Brownell, from the American University of Pennsylvania's Department of Psychiatry, summarized the phenomena well when he said that America is in the midst of an epidemic of obesity, followed by an epidemic of dieting.

The statistics in the weight loss industry are astounding. Ninety five percent (95%) of people who begin a diet to lose weight fail before they reach their goal. For the five percent (5%) that stay on their weight loss program and reach their goal, ninety percent (90%) of those gain it back within five years. (Schwartz, 1990).

WHY WEIGHT MAINTENANCE IS IMPORTANT

It is obvious that there are basic health reasons for weight control. Those who remain relatively slim have fewer health problems and are also likely to live longer. Sustaining a slender weight prevents heart disease, arthritis, diabetes, gallstones, and even cancer (Simon, 1992). It would seem reasonable to ask why on earth, with this kind of information, that obesity and weight problems remain so prevalent.

WHY MANY AMERICANS ARE OVERWEIGHT

Many of the reasons, often overlooked, is the manner in which we live our lives in modern America. When you get ready to get together with a friend, a couples, a coworker, what arrangements are most often made? Right! Let's meet for breakfast, for dinner, for lunch, for dessert. Much of our fellowship, time spent together, and getting to know one another is centered around <u>FOOD</u>.

In addition, our lifestyle tends to be about immediacy. Drive through and grab something to eat on the way to this or that. Then after that is over, why not treat yourself to an ice cream cone, or a donut, or a piece of pie. Not to mention that midst this rush through the drive-through window on the way to the next activity (which is misnamed, because "activity" normally means we are enroute to some event where we will be sitting). Who has time to schedule exercise?

Food has also become a great rewarder or comforter. I am always amazed during a normal church service when infants and toddler begin to squirm, out comes the fruit loops, the animal crackers, the suckers. When the soccer team wins, a reward is in order. And what is the reward? There is a pizza party, a weiner roast, a picnic with a bucket of chicken. When the cheerleaders do a great job, a trip to the Dairy Queen is in order. When an anniversary or a birthday rolls around, a favorite meal or dessert is prepared and served to celebrate. When a family is in grief over the sickness or loss of a loved one, we respond by taking food and goodies to their home. All of these are terrific acts of kindness. But this social habit clearly indicates our focus on <u>FOOD</u>. With this in mind, is it any wonder that we struggle so much with weight issues . . . or that 40% of American adults are obese (Berdanier et al., 1993).

With food as a major socializing issue, with weight loss programs abounding, what we often see is weight gain, weight loss, weight gained back (plus a little more), weight loss . . . and on and on. This phenomena has been called the "yo yo syndrome." *Better Nutrition for Today's Living* featured an article in the April 1994 issue that indicated "yo yo syndromes" can actually put you at greater cardiac risk and at greater risk for death than if you remained stably overweight. One of the most impactful negative consequences of "yo yo dieting" is that it changes the body's metabolism, making it more difficult to lose weight and easier to gain it back with each successive cycle of the weight gain/weight loss roller coaster (Zwiefel, 1994).

CAUSES OF OBESITY

So what is the answer to this dilemma or epidemic that plagues our nation? Researchers have been seeking answers to the cause of obesity, for new treatments for eating disorders, and for new methods to achieve and maintain weight loss. It is not surprising that thousands of studies would appear under the heading of "DHEA and Obesity" and hundreds of studies were indicated under the heading of "DHEA and Fat" when plugged into a program such as MedLine 2. Midst an avid search for natural, permanent solutions for weight loss and maintenance, DHEA has been under close scrutiny. A close review of the literature, as follows, reveals the many capacities in which DHEA could be significantly beneficial in the weight loss industry.

DHEA AND OBESITY: STUDIES IN ANIMALS

Many of the studies were conducted in a laboratory setting using animals. One of the reasons for using laboratory animals in experiments is the ease with which environments, feedings, and other conditions can be manipulated.

Speaking of studies using dogs as subjects, it may seem surprising to know that "man's best friend" is similar to man in ways you might not have expected. Earlier, it was reported that 40% of the American adult population is obese (Berdanier et al, 1993). Twenty five to fifty percent of pet dogs are also

overweight (MacEwen and Kurzman, 1991). It was determined that studying the effects of DHEA on "man's best
friend" could also reveal important information regarding its
effects in humans. Interestingly, dogs who were placed on a
high fiber diet and supplemented with DHEA lost 65.7% of
their excess body weight. Other dogs who were placed on
the same diet and given a placebo lost only 31.4% of their
body weight, indicating that DHEA and diet modification
could have as much as twice the effect as diet modification
alone (Mac Ewen and Kurzman, 1991). In another study,
Kurzman, MacEwen and Haffa (1990) found that in pets
supplemented with DHEA for three months, with no diet
modification, 68% of the dogs experienced weight loss. On
the average, they lost 4% of their total body weight per month.

FOOD DEPRIVATION NOT NECESSARY WITH DHEA TREATMENT

As mentioned earlier, most traditional weight loss programs involve some sort of modified, altered, or deprived
food intakes. If you have ever been on a "diet," as most
Americans have, you are aware of how uncomfortable and
dissatisfying these regimens can be. For many, it is a white
knuckling experience . . . "I'll do this just a few more weeks
and lose a few more pounds . . . then it will all be over and I
can eat normally again" . . . Cleary (1990) states that "long-
term success rates for treatment or prevention of obesity by
dietary intervention have been poor" (p 8). One of the reasons for the great interest in DHEA is its apparent ability to
lower body weight regardless of caloric intake.

Cleary and Zisk (1986) conducted an study using three
groups of lean and three groups of obese middle aged
femalerats. There was one group of control rats from the
lean group and one group of control rats from the obese group.
One group from the lean and one group from the obese were

supplemented orally with .6% DHEA, while the third group from each was supplemented with 1.0% DHEA. As early as the second week, both groups of obese rats being supplemented with DHEA weighed significantly less than the obese control group. There was not as much significant difference with the lean groups treated with DHEA, although they did weigh slightly less than the control group after being treated with DHEA.

This study holds the answer to a question that is asked repeatedly: "Will you just waste away after you have lost weight if you stay on DHEA?" According to this study, truly DHEA is the "mother" hormone in the sense that it knows what the body needs. The lean rats given the 1.0% DHEA lost some weight, but not excessive amounts, because there was no need for weight loss. The lean rats given .6% DHEA maintained their weight for the most part. The lean control group gained some weight in the study, which is typical of middle aged females. We all have interesting excuses for our weight gain in middle age, but even those who have been fairly lean up until middle age find weight gain begins to creep up during middle age. This study indicates that supplemental DHEA could halt some of the "middle age spread" tendencies in lean females.

In another study, obesity was induced in rats by altering diet (Mohan et. al., 1990). This compares to some of the binging that goes on in our society today. This occurs often in many of my patients and clients who starve themselves the month before going on a cruise, so that they might look just right in their new swim suit. Then while on the cruise, they eat three luscious meals a day, and return with all their previously lost weight regained . . . plus a little more.

DHEA BLOCKS THE PRODUCTION OF FAT

In this study, those rats supplemented with DHEA after

becoming obese (because of the diet they were fed), weighed less than those who were made obese, but were not treated with DHEA. Within two weeks of DHEA treatment, the diet-induced obese group weighed the same as the control group (the group that was not obesity-induced). The DHEA treatment not only blocked proliferation of new fat cells, but in addition, burned existing fat cells.

Fat loss is almost as "hot" a topic as is weight loss in our country. Since the early 1980's, people have been counting the grams of fat they consume daily, hoping to reduce their body fat. Many foods sport the "low fat" for "fat free" labels, including everything from fat-free yogurt to fat-free cookies. The body burns proteins, carbohydrates, and fats daily for energy. However, the excess is stored as body fat. The body actually prefers to store consumed fat than consumed proteins or carbohydrates. "The amount of fat you eat will ultimately determine how fat you are" (Haas, 1991, p. 37). So the increase in the attention paid to fats consumed is very critical in relation to body fat, particularly to those people desiring body fat loss.

There are two different kinds of fat in the body, brown fat and yellow fat. The brown fat serves as protection to vital organs. Yellow fat is the fat that disturbs us when we note our jeans are getting tighter than they were last year.

In 1988, a study done with normal men indicated a 31% decrease in body fat when the men were treated with DHEA (Nestler et. al, 1988). However, there was no change in body weight. Thirty one percent is an enormous decrease in the amount of fat in the human body. Particularly in men who tend to have a less overall fat content in their bodies than do females.

DHEA ACCELERATES WEIGHT LOSS

Returning to the subject of weight loss, a study with mice (Granholm et al, 1987) substantiated that as the levels of

DHEA supplemented to mice were increased, their weight gain decreased. However, not only did their weight gain decrease, but their weight loss seemed to be accelerated. I have found many males and females through the years who would be thrilled to have their weight gain stopped, and having weight loss accelerated is something that readily attracts many people's attention these days.

An additional benefit of using DHEA in weight loss is that it is not dependent on food intake (Coleman et. al, 1984). Food intake alteration seems to be a fairly unsuccessful manner of accomplishing and maintaining weight loss. Finding that DHEA does not require alterations in the food intake makes it even further desirable as a means of treating obesity. Although some studies indicate that there is a reduction of food intake in laboratory animals when DHEA is administered, this reduction is voluntary (Mohan and Cleary, 1989). Most people do not mind if their desire for food or the amount of food that they consume diminishes. However, when food intake is reduced involuntarily or due to a decision to "diet," deprivation quite often takes hold, and out of control eating begins, often in the form of binging.

A similar finding was noted in a project where different strains of rats were starved and then refed. There were significant differences in the food intake and weight gain of those rats treated with DHEA (McIntosh and Berdanier, 1988). Back during the late 1970s and early 1980s, when liquid diets were so popular, doctors remained unclear about the return of weight when some patients were put into the refeeding portion of their liquid fasting program. Perhaps the DHEA levels could have been measured and supplemented and those programs may have been more successful. Better yet, how much more preferable to lose that weight without going on weeks, months, and in some cases up to a year on liquid consumption only.

DHEA CURBS HUNGER

Another study (Mohan and Cleary, 1989) indicated that there was a reduction in food intake with rats treated with DHEA. However, it was a voluntary reduction. This study also investigated the "why's" to the weight loss accomplished with supplemental DHEA. It was noted that in the rats treated with DHEA experienced significant reductions, up to 40%, in their insulin levels. This drop in insulin levels, attributed to DHEA, could be one of the major reasons for the weight loss. Elevated insulin levels have been shown to alter metabolic efficiency, causing the body to gain weight. Once again, it is not necessary (in relation to weight loss) to test one's insulin levels. It appears that the "mother hormone" knows if these levels are off and is able to correct them spontaneously.

HOW DHEA WORKS AS AN ANTIOBESITY AGENT

There are a variety of other theories about how weight loss is actually promoted in the body with the supplementation of DHEA. One study suggests that it could be the elevated mitochondrial respiration (Mohan and Cleary, 1989); another hypothesizes that it could be due to an energy cycle involving deacylation/reacylation of fatty acyl-CoA (Cleary et al, 1984); one indicates that the weight loss is mediated by blocking the enzyme, glucose-6-phosphate dehydrogenase (G6PD) (Yen et. al, 1977); increased metabolic rate is another possible explanation (Gosnell, 1987); another study surmises that it could be because DHEA reduces dexamethasone's ability to activate tyrosine aminotransferase and ornithine decarboxylase (Wright et. al., 1992).

As you can see, the explanations for how and why DHEA impacts weight loss in the body are lengthy and complicated. As a matter of fact, in a recent workshop when some of these biochemical and biological explanations were being made, one woman spoke up and said, "Do we really have to become medical doctors to understand how this works, or can we just believe that it happens without being able to parrot the scientific explanation?"

Regardless of how or why, research clearly indicates that DHEA does aid the body in both weight and fat reduction. Scientists continue to delve into studies attempting to provide a precise explanation of how and why the weight loss and fat loss occurs. In the mean time, perhaps "it just does" is an acceptable answer. The research mentioned above, and much more, bears this out.

WHY WEIGHT LOSS IS NOT IMMEDIATE IN SOME TAKING DHEA

One study showed significantly less promising results (Usiskin et. al., 1990). Six obese men were studied for 28 days, then were supplemented with 1600 mg of DHEA daily for another 28 days. In this study, there was no significant difference in weight or body fat. However, the treatment time was shorter than other studies and the DHEA dose was less than in other studies. Once again, this indicates that some of the results of DHEA supplementation is dependent on getting enough of the DHEA in the system. It may also indicate that it may take longer than a few days or even a few weeks to see the results.

This is so difficult, because many obese and overweight people have "tried everything." When they see results, they seem more likely to stick with a program. It is much more difficult when trying a program and seeing no results immediately. Again, one of the reasons for this could also be that the "mother hormone" is finding some need in the body and is not yet working on desired weight loss or fat loss.

Fat accumulation in women has been thought to be accompanied by an increase in the adrogenic activity (Pergola et al., 1991). However, after fat accumulation continues, the adrenals may fail to keep up with the increased production it needs in order to keep weight gain and fat accumulation stopped.

According to metabolic balancing studies in the state of Washington, the adrenals, after a period of time, can be over-worked, and in a sense, can burn out. The cycle begins where demand is placed on the adrenals to produce more than they are able. This can be likened to an overworked horse. The horse may be exhausted, and the owner may need more pro-duction. The whip is then used to coax the animal to produce more, however, the energy exerted is very limited and very short lived. The same occurs with our adrenals. We may exhaust them, and then try to get them to produce more. If they are "burnt out" or exhausted, efforts are in vain.

Many dieting programs further exhaust the adrenals. However, DHEA supports and nurtures the adrenals, allow-ing the body to return to its natural ability to balance itself. When the adrenals fail to keep up with the increasing hor-mone metabolic clearance rate because of the increase in body fat mass, fat accumulation can become progressive. This is a very discouraging condition for women, and studies indicate that it can be reversed through DHEA supplementation (Per-gola et al, 1991).

When considering hormonal changes and weight gain, one of the first things to come to mind is a woman going through menopause. However, not only women are effected by hor-monal changes. In a study conducted in 1993, it was con-firmed that weight gain in men is definitely related to sex hormones (Haffner et. al., 1993). The study indicated that when the male's testosterone and oestradiol levels are down, weight tends to increase.

Obese women also have hormonal differences. Obese women tend to have normal estrone, estradiol and testosterone levels. However, their free estradiol and free testosterone levels tend to be elevated to a significant level (Zumoff, 1988). When massive weight is lost, the free estradiol and free testosterone levels then drop. Female hormones promote fat storage. This is evidenced by cattle ranchers who inject cattle with female hormones to promote rapid weight gain (Stuart and Orr, 1987, p. 31). However, the research reported throughout this chapter denotes how DHEA supplementation can act as a "mother hormone," bringing all these other hormones into balance, and promoting weight loss.

DHEA, dehydroepiandrosterone, could be one of the best kept secrets in the weight loss industry. Natural supplementation of this precursor complex could make a major difference in human health, satisfaction, and life fulfillment. More importantly, should you be one of those who have tried every weight loss program, to no avail, DHEA supplementation could be life- changing to you.

"ROCKIN' ROBBIN" NEVER FELT (OR LOOKED) BETTER!

Several days ago, a man we lovingly refer to as "Rockin' Robbin" sat in my office telling me about the vast changes in his life while taking the natural precursor products. He sat in a chair across from me, eating a granola bar in his denim shorts, and magenta shirt, absolutely glowing while telling me his story. "Rockin' Robbin" told me, when I asked how old he was, that he was 48, going on 34. . . and that really sums up his story.

He told me he came from a family where diabetes was prevalent, so doctors had been concerned for years about his glucose levels. He began taking the products about six months ago. Since that time, he has been monitored regularly by his physician. He pulled out a lab report which indicated that in the past six months, his glucose had fallen from 104 to 90;

and his triglycerides were down to 89 from 164.

He said one of his closest friends had mentioned the use of DHEA in Europe and Mexico for weight loss, but he was skeptical. He decided it was worth a try since he had been up to 232 pounds for two years. However, he could not obtain the DHEA. Later, the same friend told him about some products that were being manufactured that could be converted to DHEA in the body. So he decided skeptically to give some of the natural products a try.

Within the first month, he lost two inches in his waist. However, he only lost a couple of pounds. Tthe second month, he lost 25 pounds, believing after doing some reading about DHEA in the body that he had previously had some hormonal imbalances. He currently has lost a total of 52 pounds in six months, and has lost nine inches in his waist. He previously wore a size 42 waist, but sat in my office looking great in a pair of size 33 denim shorts.

I was congratulating him when he told me I hadn't heard the best part yet. "Rockin' Robbin" told me he had always been a slow riser, and when he did get up, he was known for his bad attitude in the mornings. He would stay in bed until the very last minute every morning, and his wife would say things like, "How on earth are you going to get up, get ready, and get to your first appointment on time?" Somehow he always did, but not without sharing his bad attitude with anyone around.

Now, he could hardly contain himself telling me how he woke up refreshed everyday, ready to get up and "get after it." He had a far superior energy level all day long, not to mention a better attitude. He said his whole family liked the difference.

I somehow couldn't imagine "Rockin' Robbin" in a blow up, but he said he had been short-fused most of his life. One of the differences he has experienced since taking the precursor complex is being less agitated and more even tempered. He was telling me how much his daughter appreciated how much better he looked, not to mention his improvement in mood, when she came in looking for him. He said, "Oh, tell her your story."

A TEENAGER IS SURPRISED WITH UNEXPECTED RESULTS

His daughter, Renee, had only begun taking the products because her dad had advised her it would just be a good health measure since it had anti-diabetic capabilities and the family had a history with diabetes. She had bought a prom dress at Christmas, and it fit perfectly, except for the length. Shortly after that, she had begun taking the products.

During spring break, she and her mom went to the tailor get the dress hemmed for prom. She slipped the dress on to be pinned, and the perfect fitting dress was all of a sudden much too large in the waist. They had expected only to have it hemmed, but they ended up removing four inches in the waist. She said: "I couldn't believe it!"

As a cheerleader, Renee said her ideal size was normally in the fall when she was the most active. Several people had told her in the winter and early spring that she looked like she had lost some weight. She said no, knowing that it just couldn't be possible with cheerleading season over. She was indeed thrilled about how her dad looks now, but she was pretty pleased with her results too.

3

DIABETES AND DHEA

Diabetes mellitus is a disease that occurs as a result of an insufficient production of insulin by the pancreas. The Greek word "diabetes" means "siphon," and the Latin word "mellitus" means "honey sweet," referring to the excess sugar in the urine. Our pancreas secretes insulin which combines with and acts on receptors located on the surfaces of our cells. The insulin tells receptors to permit sugar to enter and to let the cell use the sugar. However, if there is not enough insulin being secreted by the pancreas to send that message, the sugar begins to accumulate in the blood, then if it continues to build up, it is passed through the kidneys and is released from the body through urine.

TYPE I AND TYPE II DIABETES

There are two basic types of diabetes, Type I and Type II. Type I is sometimes called "juvenile onset" because it is normally noted at an earlier time in life than Type II. In Type I diabetes, there is such a lack of insulin in the body that insulin must be supplemented, leaving a condition known as insulin-dependent. Type II diabetes, sometimes called "maturity onset," because it is often diagnosed in adults, may be successfully treated with dietary alterations, without the use of insulin.

It is not just how sugar is metabolized in the body that is a problem for diabetics. There are also concerns with the body's utilization of fat and proteins. This is the reason for highly specialized diets among diabetics. Many of the foods in grocery stores and in some restaurants are now marked when approved by the ADA (American Diabetes Association).

INSULIN: ONCE THOUGHT A "CURE ALL"

It was once thought that insulin might be the "cure all" for diabetes and that specialized diets for the diabetics would no longer be necessary. But it was soon determined that insulin was no cure for the premature aging of vessels, so readily apparent in many diabetics. The premature aging of larger arteries cause an increased incidence of gangrene and amputations. The premature aging of the smaller arteries increases risks of blindness and kidney failure.

Except for insulin, feet are the weakest link in the diabetic. Nerve damage lessens pain sensations, and therefore, makes the diabetic more prone to foot injury. A little sore can easily become gangrenous, leading to amputation. This is a very serious concern among diabetics. The Doctors Book of Home Remedies (1990) states that once you lose a leg as a result of diabetic amputation, chances are you will lose the other one in the next three to five years (p. 1990). Diabetics are also at risk for heart disease, kidney disease, atherosclerosis, nerve damage, infection, blindness, and slow healing from cuts and bruises.

DIABETES: THE THIRD LEADING CAUSE OF DEATH

Diabetes, with its complications, is the third leading cause of death in the United States (Rector-Page, 1992, p. 196). There are approximately one million Americans diagnosed with Type II diabetes, and there are an estimated 5 million undiagnosed cases. People with diabetes are 250 times more likely than others to suffer from a stroke. Over half of diabetics die of heart disease. A study conducted at the Harvard Medical School states that diabetics are three times less likely to experience the severe pain of a heart attack than the rest of us (Berger, 1988, p. 153). Perhaps this lack of pain causes them to delay seeking treatment that is so important in coronary care.

THE IMPORTANCE OF PREVENTION

The hereditary factors of diabetes are not completely understood. The disease itself is not really what is inherited, it is the potential to develop the disease that is passed on. This is why understanding your family propensity for the disease is so critical and why early preventative treatment is essential.

THE SYMPTOMS AND CAUSES OF DIABETES

The symptoms of diabetes are high blood sugar, constant hunger with rapid, unexpected weight change, dry and itchy skin, excessive thirst, fatigue, kidney malfunction, excessive urination, blurred vision, obesity, hypertension. The symptoms of serious insulin deprivation can be anything from mental confusion to a coma (Nyholt, 1993, p. 55).

The causes of diabetes are varied. They include such things as: poor diet with too many refined foods, fats and carbohydrates; insulin, chromium, and HCI deficiencies; glucose and fat metabolism malfunction, leading to obesity; pancreas and liver malfunction due to excessive caffeine, alcohol, and or stress; heredity factors; hypothyroidism. Diabetes can also occur in pregnant women, but is usually normalized as soon as the baby is born. Some drugs, such as blood pressure medication, some hormonal prescription drugs, and some drugs used to treat psychiatric conditions can cause the onset of diabetes. Dietary patterns can also cause the onset of the condition.

BEING CAUTIOUS AND SELF TREATMENT

In most of the chapters in this book, there are many of recommendations to consider about natural treatments and supplementation of vitamins, herbs, exercise and other such holistic approaches. It is so imperative to stress with diabetics that supplementing with anything should be done with the approval of and close monitoring by their physician.

Diabetics and their doctors might consider Chromium GTF (glucose tolerance factor) as a supplemental treatment as it may enhance the effect of insulin. Niacin, one of the B Vitamins, can help potentiate the effects of chromium. Inositol protects nerves from the damage they often suffer due to the high sugar levels in diabetics. Anthocyanic acid has been shown to lower blood sugar in some cases. Vitamin C helps fight infections and heal wounds, an important concern to diabetics. Magnesium is important in cell production and is lost frequently through the urine of diabetics. Vitamin B1 is very important in the process of metabolizing sugar. Garlic suppresses yeast. Diabetics tend to get more yeast infections because yeast thrives in high sugar environments. "Garlic is one of the few completely harmless natural substances which are effective in the treatment of diabetes" (Airola, 1982, p. 81). Acidophilus is also helpful in the high sugar environment because it keeps the intestinal flora from yeast multiplication.

As mentioned earlier, one of the most important aspects in diabetes is preventative treatment. Many times some of the premature aging of the arteries is done before the condition is actually diagnosed. Therefore, noting family history, and becoming engaged in preventative measures, is a key factor in long-term health.

DHEA AS AN ANTIDIABETES AGENT

Once again, we can turn to the vast research on DHEA and find great hope for those with familial diabetes. One of the important facts to note about age and diabetes is that it is characterized by the cell's loss of sensitivity to insulin. In a study, using diabetic mice, it was shown that DHEA acted in insulin resistant mice to increase their sensitivity to insulin (Coleman et. al., 1984). The same study noted that early, preventative DHEA treatment with these same mice prevented the development of most of the symptoms of diabetes. In a study using rats, fasting insulin levels were not altered in lean rats, but were significantly lower in obese, diabetic rats treated with DHEA (Cleary et. al., 1988). Coleman (1990) also found that DHEA reduced blood sugar concentrations to normal.

Several recent studies found that DHEA improved insulin sensitivity (Buffington, et.al., 1993; Cleary, 1990; Mohan et.al., 1990). The reasons that this might be true is that DHEA is a precursor for estrogen and testosterone. However, the estrogens are more potent in their ability to block diabetes in mice (Coleman et.al., 1982, p. 833). When DHEA was given to these mice, they produced more estrogen than lean mice to which they were compared. Another study demonstrated that the condition of hyperinsulinemia, too much insulin in the body, may decrease DHEA and DHEAS levels, which then promote atherosclerotic processes (Nestler Et.Al., 1992). They suggest that DHEA may be the "missing link" between hyperinsulinemia and atherosclerotic, implying that DHEA may be supplemented to prevent some of the premature aging of the arteries so typical in diabetics.

DiaBeta and Micronase, two of the most common drugs prescribed to treat diabetes, have been shown to increase death rates from heart disease. However, DHEA has been shown to decrease the risk of cardiovascular disease (see chapter on cardiovascular disease).

Although you should check with your physician before making any changes in your diet and/or medication, and before adding even a natural precursor hormone, DHEA could be a giant step in preventing diabetes and in treating the symptoms of diabetes.

A SUCCESS STORY FROM A PHYSICIAN

A good friend of mine, whom I will call Ann, is a doctor in a small community outside of a major metropolitan area. About four years ago, she was diagnosed with diabetes. She first tried taking some of the oral agents, however, they did not control her symptoms. She then had to begin taking 30 units of insulin in the morning and 30 more each evening. A mutual friend of ours told her about some of the natural precursor products to DHEA, and as a doctor, Ann was already aware of the many benefits of DHEA. She got some of the natural products and began taking them. After three months, she has been able to reduce her insulin to 20 units in the morning and 20 in the evening. She hopes to be able to continue to back off of it. Another pleasant victory Ann told me about on the phone recently is the fact that she has dropped two dress sizes in the process as well! She also is recommending the natural precursor products to her patients.

4

THE CARDIOVASCULAR SYSTEM AND THE POWERFUL EFFECTS OF DHEA

The human cardiovascular system is a marvel of engineering and fluid mechanics. The heart is a powerful muscular organ pumping blood through a system of chambers and valves into the circulatory system for distribution to the body. Our tough and resilient heart muscle is very busy, pumping the 22 trillion blood cells in our five quarts of blood throughout our body. In 70 years, the heart beats more than 2.5 billion times and pumps some 165 million quarts of blood.

This vital organ is about the size of a clenched fist and weighs a little more than half a pound. From the intricate capillaries at the extreme edge of the circulatory system, nutrients and oxygen enter all cells of the body, and then the waste products of metabolism are transferred into the blood.

The heart is made up of four chambers. The top two chambers, called atria, are thin-walled reservoirs that distend to collect blood as it pours in from the veins between beats. The lower two chambers, called ventricles, are thick-walled pumping chambers that receive blood from the upper chambers and drive it into the arteries. (It is this drive that creates what we call a "heartbeat). The right two chambers receive oxygen-poor blood from the body and push it into the lungs. The left two chambers receive oxygenated blood from the lungs and push it into the body. Because of the great work it must perform, the left ventricle is by far the thickest and heaviest chamber of the heart.

THE PREVALENCE OF CORONARY DISEASE

Cardiovascular disease is the most prevalent degenerative disease known to mankind. In the U.S. alone it is the underlying cause of nearly 750,000 deaths each year. People are really just as old (or as young) as their arteries are. This disease is of great public health concern in America. Premature death and disability cause enormous physical and emotional suffering, as well as significant economic losses. Our society is constantly searching for ways to improve our cardiovascular health.

OUR HEART'S GREATEST ENEMY: ATHEROSCLEROSIS

The great enemy of our cardiovascular system is atherosclerosis. Atherosclerosis is a thickening of the interior linings of our arteries that can lead to obstruction of blood flow. Fatigue, angina, and strokes are the result of this obstruction.

CARDIOVASCULAR HEALTH

The major lifestyle components of cardiovascular health are well known: don't smoke, exercise regularly, eat a diet of fruits and vegetables and low fat foods. However, getting people to change the way they live, even if it makes a great difference in the quality of their lives, has proven to be an extremely difficult task. The search for other protective measures continues unabated. The use of some antioxidants, like Vitamin E and beta carotene have gained widespread acceptance. Perhaps the use of DHEA, in a natural form, will become one of those generally accepted protective measures someday.

DHEA LEVELS AND HEART DISEASE

The connection between DHEA and heart disease is striking. Study after study has shown a direct correlation between DHEA (and DHEA - Sulfate) and lower incidence of heart disease. The particular relationship between cardiac and circulatory system function and DHEA has been explored in numerous projects, in many ways, including: tissue culture studies, animal studies, and human clinical and population studies. An attempt will be made in this chapter to summarize the findings of these various studies.

SEX-RELATED DIFFERENCES

Sex differences in the blood concentrations of DHEA become observable at puberty and continue as we age (de Perritti, et.al., 1973). Young girls have higher levels of DHEA than young boys (Anderson, et.al., 1976). Another study found higher concentrations of DHEA in male subjects under 45 years of age than in females in the same age group (Hopper, et.al., 1975). Several other studies have shown higher metabolic conversion rates and different excretory rates for females as compared to males (Bird, C.E., et.al., 1984). Metabolic studies indicate that the way DHEA is eliminated also differs in males and females. Females excrete more androsterone and etiocholanolonethan males. In addition, females convert a much greater portion of their DHEA into a sulfate than males. Since cardiovascular disease rates are the highest in males at every age level, this is of significant interest. One conclusion that could be drawn from this is that female-male differences in DHEA levels may explain why there are some of the sex differences in the association of blood concentrations and DHEA with cardiovascular disease. It is possible, however, that the association of DHEA sulfate to cardiovascular disease in males, but not in females, is related to a deficiency of DHEA in males (Barrett-Conner, et.al., 1986).

DIFFERENCES IN DHEA LEVELS ABOUT DIFFERENT RACES

For decades, public health officials and researchers have speculated about the source of racial differences in cardiovascular disease. Possible genetic differences in disease susceptibility have been postulated.

Significant racial differences in blood levels of DHEA sulfate have been found in geographically distinct populations. The DHEA sulfate levels were 10 to 20% higher in adult Caucasian females in England than Japanese females of the same menopausal status (Wang, et.al., 1976). Caucasian British males had DHEA sulfate levels that were twice as high as black Kenyan males (Wang, et.al., 1968).

AGE, CARDIOVASCULAR DISEASE AND DHEA LEVELS

The relationship between age and cardiovascular disease is well known. Age-related differences in DHEA levels are consistently noted in human population studies, and are referenced in throughout this book. Some researchers speculate that declining DHEA levels may be one of the physiologic mechanisms of aging. Because of these relationships, age must be considered when examining the relationship between DHEA and cardiovascular health. Again, most studies show an inverse association between DHEA blood levels and age, meaning, the older we get, the lower our DHEA levels become (Zumoff, B., et.al., 1980). Studies show a distinctive decline in the blood levels of DHEA Sulfate with each passing decade after the 30s (Orentreich, et.al., 1984).

CARDIOVASCULAR RISK AND DHEA

The levels of lipids in the blood are well known predictors for the development of cardiovascular disease. Watching the cholesterol level is a favorite pastime for many health-conscious Americans (see chapter on Cholesterol). The association of the levels of lipids in the blood and DHEA is of keen interest.

In a cross-sectional study of 554 adults with 236 men and 318 women, measuring serum DHEA and DHEA sulfate in each, DHEA was shown to be positively correlated with high density lipoprotein (HDL) cholesterol, the "good cholesterol" in men. However, the same was not true for women. The same study revealed that low density lipoprotein (LDL) cholesterol, the "bad cholesterol", and triglycerides were inversely associated with DHEA sulfate in women but not in men (Nafziger, et.al., 1990).

Another study, examining 204 heart disease patients being prepared to have a coronary angiography, found DHEA sulfate directly associated with LDL. The higher the LDL levels, the lower the DHEA levels. This study was adjusted for age differences and the level differences commonly associated with those differences. This is important because blood cholesterol concentrations are usually higher with increasing age. Conversely, levels of DHEA tend to move lower with age. The fact that these studies indicate an association between DHEA sulfate and cholesterol levels is made even stronger because of its persistence after an age adjustment (Herrington, et.al., 1990).

SMOKING, CARDIOVASCULAR DISEASE AND DHEA

The relationship between smoking and cardiovascular disease is one of the strongest environment-related health risks ever identified. It is the most important modifiable risk factor in our culture. Given the general direction of virtually all studies regarding the health aspects of DHEA, the studies on DHEA and smoking are really surprising. Studies have found significantly higher concentrations of DHEA sulfate in smokers of both sexes when compared with nonsmokers. This is true even after the adjustments are made for age and body mass index (Herrington et.al., 1990, Khaw, et.al., 1988). Researchers speculate that the higher levels of DHEA are caused by nicotine's stimulating ACTH release, which in turn causes increases in DHEA production. A partial adrenal enzymatic block causing lower conversion rates of DHEA sulfate to other sulfates has been postulated. Given the population-wide reduction of cardiovascular disease associated with higher DHEA levels, it would seem the evidence about smokers means an even more significant and positive relationship than would otherwise appear to be true.

STRESS AND DHEA

The relationship between stress and DHEA levels has been reported, particularly those stresses that are associated with medical concerns. The studies focus on medical concerns and stresses because blood concentrations of various kinds are measured for other medical reasons, and the DHEA levels were simply added to gather additional data. Serious medical stress, such as that associated with having a major surgery, having a heart attack, or the significant worsening of a chronic illness, are all associated with decreases in levels of DHEA. After an apparent initial jump in the production of all steroid-type hormones, possibly because of the release of adrenalin, our fight or flight hormone, steroid metabolism shifts to the increased production of glucocorticoids and away from androgens, including DHEA (Parker, et.al., 1985, Yamaji, 1969).

TYPE A BEHAVIOR AND DHEA

Another of the more interesting studies of cardiovascular risk factors focused on what is known as "Type A" behavior. Type A behavior is characterized by high levels of aggression, hostility, and competitiveness. Although not clearly established, this type of behavior has been associated with increased cardiovascular disease. One review hypothesized an inverse relation of Type A behavior with DHEA. The reviewer postulated that exaggerated glucocorticoid responses was linked to hypersecretion of cortisol and decreased secretion of DHEA Sulfate. If this cause-effect relationship exists, the study suggested this mechanism could explain lower levels of DHEA associated with both acute stress and Type A behavior patterns.

DHEA AND ATHEROSCLEROSIS

The relationship between DHEA and atherosclerosis has been the subject of a considerable number of investigations. One large study considered the relationship between DHEA sulfate concentrations and subsequent 12-year cardiovascular and ischemic heart disease mortality in 242 men, aged 50 to 79 years. (Ischemia is a condition characterized by a decrease in the blood supply to some part of the body. Ischemic heart disease refers to a decrease in the supply of blood getting to the heart. It is often accompanied by pain, and sometimes by organ dysfunction. Some causes of ischemic heart disease are arterial embolism, atherosclerosis, thrombosis, and vasoconstriction). The study reported that at lower DHEA levels of less than 100 mg/dl, the cardiovascular mortality rates per 100 persons were 20.4. When DHEA levels were 110-179 mg/dl, the mortality rates per 100 persons was 15.0. Finally, when the DHEA levels were 180 mg/dl, the mortality rate was reduced to 6.8 per 100 persons. This study also found there was a dose response relation. Ater this study was reported, a report on additional subjects from the same population was published. It found the same inverse association between DHEA sulfate and death rates due to cardiovascular disease in men (Barrett, et.al., 1986).

VARIOUS STUDIES ABOUT CARDIOVASCULAR DISEASE AND DHEA

A study was conducted using 103 women and 103 men who were about to undergo coronary angiography. The study found a significant inverse association between DHEA sulfate levels and the extent of angiographically defined coronary artery disease in men but not in women. In women, DHEA was found not to be associated with coronary artery stenosis (constriction or narrowing of the artery). When adjusted for conventional cardiovascular risk factors (smoking, total cholesterol, HDL and LDL cholesterol, age, cholesterol triglycerides, and diabetes), DHEA was shown to have an independent association with coronary heart disease in men. The sex differences have been attributed to the fact that at the time of coronary angiography, women tend to have less extensive disease compared with men. The differences in DHEA association in women could be secondary to a decrease in the power to find such an association because of less extensive disease (Murdaugh, et.al., 1988).

One study compared four groups of men: men six months after myocardial infarction (blockage of an artery); men with angiograms showing disease; men with angiograms showing no disease; and normal controls. The results were significant. Men who already had myocardial infarctions had the highest blood concentrations of DHEA, and the normal controls had the lowest. Men with angiograms showing heart disease had DHEA concentrations lower than those men who had previous infarctions, and higher than the men without

disease showing in angiograms. The authors of the study
suggested that higher blood concentrations of DHEA predis-
pose men to survival after myocardial infarction (Zumoff
et.al., 1982).

Two studies investigated the levels of several steroid concentrations directly. The higher concentrations found in most
studies suggest that a decrease in clearance and/or metabolism of DHEA may be present in subjects with cardiovascular disease. These studies are consistent with myocardial
infarction survivorship. (Zumoff, et.al., 1982; Slowinska-
Srednicka, 1989).

ADMINISTERING DHEA
TO CARDIOVASCULAR PATIENTS

Several studies have investigated the exogenous (from
outside the body) administration of DHEA on the effects on
cardiovascular disease or its risk factors. In nine case reports
of either angina or intermittent claudication (cramp-like pains
in the calf muscles caused by poor circulation in the leg
muscles), each patient reported significant relief from symptoms from administration of oral DHEA. Alleviation of sever
angina was reported in three elderly men after taking DHEA.
One subject experienced a complete resolution of ischemic
electrocardiographic changes (Fassati, et.al., 1970). The quick
responses found in these case studies with relief from angina
indicate that the positive effects of DHEA was not only due
to reversal of atherosclerosis. There was just not enough time
for that to occur. So in addition to DHEA's ability to reverse
atherosclerosis, it obviously has some other positive effects
on cardiovascular disease.

In a random cross-over trial, six healthy women received
DHEA or a placebo for four weeks. An 11% decline in cholesterol was observed within just one week of the supplementation of the DHEA, with a 20% decrease in HDL cho-

lesterol (Mortola, et.al., 1990). This is another important study to support the idea that DHEA may be an effective treatment for, or at least a preventative of, cardiovascular disease.

CONCLUSIONS ABOUT DHEA
AND CARDIOVASCULAR DISEASE

The studies referenced here, plus many others not specifically cited, provide a great layman's insight into the striking relationship between DHEA and the cardiovascular system. The relations between blood lipids (cholesterol) and cardiovascular risk is well established. Studies have shown that DHEA can influence synthesis of fatty acids, cholesterol, and phospholipids. A direct association of DHEA and HDL cholesterol has been shown in men, but not in women. This may explain some of the sex differences in the positive effects of DHEA on cardiovascular disease.

Studies show DHEA to be effective in lessening the impact of diabetes. Researchers postulate even more significant benefits with controlled administration of DHEA. Prevention and/or moderation of diabetes in humans by both naturally-occuring or administered DHEA needs further study. Administration of DHEA has shown immunosuppression activity in relation to insulin production in mice. The relation of naturally occurring DHEA to immunologic processes should be studied further.

Studies show that DHEA may regulate fat metabolism, the size of fat deposit, and its distribution. Links between obesity and DHEA have been shown. Researchers suggest that DHEA may be the hormonal link between obesity and increased risk of cardiovascular disease.

Further study of the relation between androgen and estrogen metabolism may shed light on the sex differences in cardiovascular disease. Studies point to a DHEA hormonal role in atherosclerosis. The mechanisms of this activity are not clearly known at this time, but speculation regarding cell-level effects, particularly in artery wall construction, should lead to some further studies in the future.

It can be stated with certainty that studies to date point to DHEA's signirficant protective role in cardiovascular disease. The data suggests that higher levels of DHEA in the circulatory system, particularly in men, protects against the occurrence of such diseases. The data is not as strong for women, but several researchers have provided explanations for this phenomenon. It is possible that research methodology causes some of the sex differences. Biologic action of DHEA may actually provide some of the explanation for sex differences in cardiovascular disease in general.

Sifting through the studies, Anne Nafziger and her group (1991) postulate that further research may reveal two different and distinct subgroups within the human population. One group may consist of smokers and those with high saturated fat diets. This group may have high levels of DHEA sulfate and an increased incidence of cardiovascular disease. The incidence of their disease is a result of these negative lifestyles, and overrides any other considerations. The second group may consist of those with decreased adrenal function, diabetes, and obesity. They may have low levels of DHEA sulfate and an increased incidence of cardiovascular disease. Increased levels of DHEA may or may not help individuals with these health problems.

It is clear that a tremendous amount of research on the relationship between DHEA on cardiovascular disease needs to be done. The effect of many disease-related factors, such as smoking, estrogen use, and hypertension, must be isolated and determined. Research to date provides some significant first clues as to the importance of DHEA and cardiovascular. This evidence must be pursued.

A "HEART-FELT" STORY

One delightful young lady, whom I will call D'Ann came bubbling in my office recently. She was telling a story to one of the people out front. I couldn't quite hear, but the energy level was so high that I had to stick my head out of my office.

D'Ann was telling a story, laughing, smiling, and crying . . . all at the same time. Her dad had bypass surgery a little more than 10 years ago. Apparently, he had not been doing well for several months, and D'Ann was worried. His constant fatigue left the family worried that another bypass surgery would follow soon.

D'Ann had heard my lecture about the research on cardiovascular disease and benefits of DHEA. She had asked where to get the natural precursor complex products made from the Wild Mexican Yam, Dioscorea. She then asked her dad to try them.

Not only was her dad better, but he had called from a vacation with her mom that day, had walked all over the airport, and hadn't felt better in years. With tears, thanking God, D'Ann had stopped by to thank us for the lecture, for directing her to products that could help her aging father.

Recently, I called D'Ann's home, and her dad answered the phone. He recognized my name and thanked me again for directing his daughter to something so beneficial. In the conversation, he told me that his wife, who had hereditary fatty knots on her arms for 30 years, and had some surgically removed, was more than thrilled. She took the products just for health measures, and much to her surprise, all the knots had disappeared!

In a society of high stress, fast foods, and sedentary lifestyles, it is certainly in our best interest to do what we are able to do to prevent ourselves and our loved ones from cardiovascular disease.

5

MENOPAUSE, HORMONE REPLACEMENT THERAPY, AND OSTEOPOROSIS: DHEA TO THE RESCUE

"Menopause – Nature's course correction when a woman no longer has to put up with the nuisance of monthly periods, free to exercise her lusty libido without the risk of pregnancy and the burden of bearing children, a time when she is likely freed of child care, still in good health, and full of the wisdom of life. What a blessed gift of Mother Nature!" (Lee, 1993, p. 31). I am not sure that many women view the "change of life" in such a glamorous way.

Although we traditionally have women in mind when we use the word menopause, there are many writers who believe that men experience a similar "change of life." In a woman's life, the changes are fairly obvious as she experiences changes in her menstrual cycle. Dr. Smith (1989) believes that because men do not have a marked physiological occurrence in their bodies, their "change" could be more confusing. He believes it is during this time in a man's life that there is confusion, depression, and a personal crisis of emotions. He suggests that this "change" can be manifested in many forms: emotional explosions, confusing feelings, irritability, reversion to adolescent behaviors (promiscuity, fatigue, acne), depression, back problems, indigestion. Clearly, both men and women go through some physiological and emotional changes and challenges as they approach their fifth decade of life.

WHAT IS MENOPAUSE?

Menopause is a time in a woman's life when her ovaries cease functioning, her estrogen secretion slows down, and her monthly menstrual bleeding ceases. The word menopause is taken from two Greek words: "mens" which means monthly and "pausa" which means stop. The average age of menopause in the United States is about age 49.8. For active smokers, the age is 48.13. For passive smokers, those married to or living with an active smoker, the average age is 49.1. Interestingly, menopause occurs significantly earlier in left-handed women (Kamen, 1993). Menopause also can be induced by surgical removal of the ovaries much earlier. Approximately a half a million American women have hysterectomies annually (Nyholt, 1993).

THE SYMPTOMS OF MENOPAUSE

Perhaps the words "the change" refer to the time when hormonal changes brings about physiological and emotional "changes" in a woman's life. The drop in production of estrogen and progesterone in the ovaries can have a profound effect on mood, energy level, bone mineralization, temperature regulation, and libido. Actually, the term menopause refers to the time when the actual cyclical bleeding halts. The time most often referred to as "the change", when symptoms are abounding, is called the perimenopausal cycle. The symptoms are many and varied and include such complaints as: irregular periods, hot flashes, hot flushes, depression, aches, pains, difficulty breathing, dizziness, headaches, heart palpitations, dry skin, vaginal dryness, emotional instability, insomnia, stiffening or aching joints, sore breasts, abdominal congestion (constipation, gas, bloating), night sweats, mood changes, vaginal discomfort, not feeling oneself, outbursts of anger, thinking in slow motion, tingling hands and feet, numb sensations in hands and feet, chills, fluctuating sexual interest, painful intercourse, urinary tract infections and leakage, loss of pubic and underarm hair.

All these symptoms vary in occurrence and severity individual to individual. The can last anywhere from several months to several years. According to Gladstar (1993), approximately 10% of women experience none of these symptoms; approximately 80% experience some of the symptoms, but find them tolerable; and approximately 10% express discomfort or disturbance about the symptoms. Lee (1993) believes that approximately 50 to 60% of women go through menopause symptom-free.

Dr. Rector-Page states it well: "Menopause is intended by nature to be a gradual reduction of estrogen by the ovaries with few side effects. In a well-nourished, vibrant woman, the adrenals and other glands pick up the job of estrogen secretion to keep her active and attractive after menopause" (1992, p. 271). Perhaps the reason this transition doesn't always occur as easily is the "ungraceful aging" we experience due to our "ungraceful" lifestyle. Our poor eating habits, stressful way of living, and the lack of exercise, certainly is a setup for "ungraceful aging" (Gladstar, 1993).

ONCE UPON A TIME
ELDERLY WOMEN WERE HONORED

In traditional cultures, older women were honored as village elders and were held in a place of reverence and respect. In these cultures, menopause was not the "curse" that it is traditionally seen today. New attitudes toward the elderly are almost contemptuous. Particularly for elderly women. Somehow, as men develop wrinkles around their eyes, graying at their temples, he is held as "distinguished" or "wise."

Yet women, who are valued for youth, beauty, and sex, do not receive the same place of honor as they age. They are "traded in for younger models" . . . Then it is wondered why this change is an emotional experience.

Gladstar (1993, p. 208) suggests that "if we can change self-image and attitudes, this moment in our lives can be an empowering, celebratory rite of passage as indeed it should be." It is a shame that a time many women look forward to, free of responsibilities, children, periods, can become so confusing. Anthropologist Margaret Mead refers to menopause as PMZ – postmenopausal zest – a time when women, unencumbered by pregnancies and periods are finally <u>FREE</u>! Perhaps one way to ensure it is a celebratory time is to understand what to expect, how to cope with it, and to grasp a positive mindset about the whole experience.

Calculation of Menopausal Distress

Each menopausal symptom is listed with a given "factor." In the column head "Severity," enter the number that reflects the severity of your current experience: 0 for none, 1 for slight, 2 for moderate, and three for heavy. Then multiply your severity score by the listed factor to fill in the numerical conversion.

When you add up the numerical conversion column, you will have a score known as the Kupperman Menopausal Index. If your score is more than 35, you have severe menopausal symptoms. If your score is less than 20, your symptoms are mild.

Symptom	Factor	X	Severity (0-3)	=	Numerical Conversion
Hot flashes/night sweats	4	X	_____	=	_____
Prickling/burning	2		_____		_____
Insomnia	2		_____		_____
Nervousness	2		_____		_____
Melancholia (Depression)	1		_____		_____
Vertigo (Dizziness)	1		_____		_____
Weakness (Fatigue)	1		_____		_____
Muscle/joint pain	1		_____		_____
Headache	1		_____		_____
Palpitation	1		_____		_____
Formication	1		_____		_____
(Itchy feeling on the skin)					

Kupperman Menopausal Index Total   _____

The previous chart, called the Kupperman Menopausal Index, (taken from Dr. Cutler's *Hysterectomy: Before and After*, 1988) can help you to determine the severity of the symptoms experienced during menopause.

If you have mild symptoms, you will still want to read this chapter to be more educated about the symptoms and their treatments! If you discover that your struggle with symptoms is severe, you will find the information in the rest of this chapter helpful to you in coping with this time in your life.

HOT FLASHES AND FLUSHES

Hot flashes are experienced by 75% of women experiencing menopause (Gladstar, 1993). These are called flushes, flushings, and sweats. They can last from one or two seconds to several minutes. However long the actual flash may last, it can take up to half an hour for your body to feel normalized once the flash has occurred. There are several hypotheses about why these hot flashes occur. One is vasomotor instability which affects nerve centers and blood flow, creating a hot sensation. A second is the pituitary may increase production of ovary stimulating hormone when it senses the ovary's production of estrogen and progesterone is down, creating a glandular imbalance. The hot flash may actually be the body's attempt to balance itself hormonally. A third theory is that the hormonal changes may irritate blood vessels and nerves, causing them to overdilate, producing a hot feeling.

SWELLING AND BLOATING

Another common symptom is that of water retention. Hormones, and most especially estrogen, regulates the balance of fluid in our bodies. When estrogen fluctuates, the body's sodium levels increase, causing our cells to retain more water. Even the retention of a few ounces of water can cause a substantial difference in our bodies, such as: breast tenderness, depression, bloating, anxiety, back aches. These back aches can be treated with valerian root or hot herbal baths of pennyroyal, lavender or chamomile herbs (Gladstar, 1993). When our bodies begin to retain fluids and we notice we cannot get that ring on our finger, our first reaction is to limit our intake of fluid. This is, in fact, the opposite of the response we need to have. We need to increase our intake of fluids, avoids salts, and definitely, stay away from diuretics!

VAGINAL DRYNESS

Vaginal dryness (atropic vaginitis) is also one of the common symptoms of menopause. This dryness occurs due to a thinning of the vaginal lining. The mucous membranes begin to thin, causing a loss in the elasticity of the vaginal walls. Vaginal dryness is often the key reason stated by physicians for estrogen replacement therapy, however, often vaginal dryness can be overcome by using the Kegel exercises, developed by Dr. Kegel in the 1940s. The exercise basically involved exercising the PC muscle (the pubococcygeus). This is the muscle used to stop urination. You simply practice tightening and releasing that muscle, working up to 200 times daily. This exercise strengthens the muscle, drawing fresh blood into vaginal tissue, which assists in creating thicker vaginal walls, which are more moist.

ADDRESSING MENOPAUSE AND HORMONAL IMBALANCES WITH MOTHER NATURES' TREATMENTS

There are many ideas about natural treatment regimens for menopause and its variety of symptoms. One is eating foods high in calcium and iron, such as: cottage cheese, spinach, lobster, spaghetti, beets, apricots, whole grains, bran, raisins, molasses, sunflower seeds. Vitamins D, C, B complex, B6 are all recommended (Lauersen and Stukane, 1983). Herbal recommendations include: ginseng (to relieve hot flashes), dong quai (to alleviate vaginal dryness), vitex, black cohosh, fennel (Lee, 1993 and Mindell, 1992). Gladstar (1993) recommends making teas, tonics, and tablets containing the Wild Yam extract, as well as supplementing with bee pollen and spirulina.

One of the most natural, and most helpful natural treatments, is exercise. Exercise is essential in strengthening our bones. Any exercise – walking, biking, weight lifting, can be beneficial, but swimming may be one of the most beneficial to menopausal women because it never places a strain on her bones. "Both the production and use of hormones are maximized by sufficient activity" (Gladstar, 1993, p. 215).

HORMONAL PRODUCTION THROUGH MENOPAUSE

As stated earlier, menopause is a time when the ovaries slow down, then cease, their production of hormones. However, this does not mean that the body is all of a sudden without any of these hormones at all. In a healthy woman, with a healthy adrenal system, the adrenals take over the sex hormone production. The healthier your adrenals are, the less likely you will experience the unpleasant symptoms of menopause. Unfortunately, many females have worn out their adrenals by the time they reach menopause and therefore, the adrenals are not able to help them out at a time when they are needed. Adrenal stress is many times the result of extreme stress for long period of time. It is known by symptoms such as: nervous disorders, unpredictable mood swings, fatigue, irritability, severe depression. You can imagine that if your adrenal system is worn out and already has some of these symptoms, and then your body begins to call upon it to supplement the production of sex hormones, that it can certainly send out messages of exhaustion through the above listed symptoms. Perhaps this is the reason for the severity of menopausal symptoms in some women.

STRENGTHENING AND NOURISHING YOUR ADRENAL SYSTEM

Regardless, the years before and during menopause are definitely a time to nourish your adrenal health. This can be done by providing your body with plenty of oxygen through a regular exercise program and by developing some deep breathing exercises. Exercise programs not only provide extra oxygen to the adrenals, but it also relieves the body of stress, which places natural wear and tear on the adrenals. Deep breathing exercises relieve one of stress, as well as provide extra oxygen to the adrenals. One deep breathing exercise that can be practiced regularly is to inhale through the nostrils to a slow count of five, hold the breath to a slow count of twenty, and then exhale through the mouth to a slow count of ten. This exercise should be repeated at least ten times daily to begin strengthening the adrenals. Supplements that can bolster the adrenal system are: Vitamin C, B5, magnesium, Siberian ginseng, ginseng, Indian ginseng, licorice and tumeric.

HORMONAL REPLACEMENT: PROS AND CONS

There are some ways to supplement the hormones, progesterone and estrogen, as their levels drop. The debate has been which ones to supplement, how much, and whether to supplement with natural and/or synthetics. One might wonder, with all this debate, if Mother Nature made a mistake by allowing progesterone deficiencies to occur in women around menopause? It is interesting to note that in other cultures, the deficiencies do not occur. Dr. Lee (1993) indicates that the mistake is not with Mother Nature, but with our advanced lifestyles. There are over 5,000 plants that make sterols that can convert to estrogen and progesterone. However, our culture turns to processed foods, foods that are treated with chemicals, foods that are picked long before they reach our stores, and then our homes. By this time, their vitamin and sterol levels have dropped dramatically, and we end up consuming empty calories.

Before entering a discussion about estrogen replacement, it is important to know that the term "estrogen" refers to a class of hormones with estrus activity (Lee, 1993). There are actually three different classes: El (estrone) and E2 (estradiol) when supplemented are the two that increase the risk of breast cancer. E3 (estriol) is the estrogen most prominent in pregnant women and serves as a protector from breast cancer. So when estrogen replacement is considered, estriol is the one best for supplementation.

In 1979, Dr. Hammond and his associates conducted a study over a five year period to determine the long term effects when estrogen replacement therapy was used. The positive effects noted were: lower rates of coronary disease, lower occurrences of hypertension and osteoporosis. The detrimental effects noted included: increased uterine bleeding and increased risk of endometrial cancer (1979).

In reviewing the literature, Dr. Hargrove and his associates noted the above stated benefits of estrogen replacement therapy, but also noted that estrogen replacement therapy prevented genital atrophy (1989). According to Dr. Felson and his associates, who published a study in The New England Journal of Medicine in October of 1993, seven years of estrogen replacement therapy is needed to provide a long term protective effect on bone mineral density. Then, even with that seven years, it may not protect women over 75.

The arguments against estrogen replacement therapy abound. Although it seems to be a "pie in the sky" resolution for many physicians dealing with menopausal women, there are serious side effects. Gladstar (1993) points to the seriousness of the risks for cancer of the endometrial lining of the uterus with estrogen replacement therapy. The average occurrence of endometrial cancer in postmenopausal women in 1 in 1,000. However, for those who have been on estrogen replacement therapy for two to four years, the percentages for those at risk increase 4 to 8 times. For those who have been on the therapy for seven or more years, the percentages of risk increase 14 times. In addition to this serious concern, Gladstar (1993) lists other side effects of estrogen replacement therapy: water retention, weight gain, breast tenderness, depression, excessive mood swings, and an increase in size of benign tumors of the uterus. This certainly substantiates a look at the opinions and research of those who oppose estrogen replacement therapy.

Dr. John Lee of Sebastopol, California, strongly states his opinion: "Many postmenopausal women do not need estrogen replacement. Not only does a woman's body continue to produce some estrogen but she is ingesting phytoestrogens (estrogenic substances found in plants) and is exposed to xenoestrogens (estrogenic substances of petrochemical origin in the environment). The addition of progesterone enhances the receptors of estrogen and thus her 'need' for estrogen may not exist" (1993). Dr. Lee's preceding statement introduces another topic: unopposed estrogens. Unopposed estrogen is a term used to describe estrogen replacement therapy given without supplementation of progesterone.

The Lancet published an article in 1990 which examined estrogen/progestagen hormonal replacement therapy. It stated that unopposed estrogens cause endometrial hyperstimulation which leads to irregular vaginal bleeding, endometrial hyperplasia, and cancer. They also stated that the cancer risk persisted fifteen years after the estrogen replacement therapy was terminated (Whitehead et. al., 1990). A study conducted at the Boston University School of Medicine determined that women who used estrogen without progesterone had a 6.5 times greater risk of developing endometrial cancer than women who did not use estrogen replacement. They also found that women who combined estrogen replacement therapy with progesterone did not have any increase in risk of cancer (Donaldson, 1993).

HORMONAL REPLACEMENT: SYNTHETIC OR NATURAL?

If estrogen replacement therapy should be accompanied by progesterone, the next debate is whether synthetic or natural hormone supplementation should be used. Dr. Hargrove and his associates noted in their study that synthetic estrogen exaggerated potency in the hepatic system and that synthetic estrogens reduce the benefits that estrogen is reported to have on the cardiovascular system (Hargrove et.al., 1989). This study showed natural supplements preferable to synthetics: "We and others have demonstrated that a micronized natural progesterone preparation administered orally can produce excellent blood levels without the unwanted effects (such as fluid retention, breast tenderness, weight gain, and depression of the synthetics" (Hargrove et. al, 1989, p. 607). In their study, they had a group of women they treated with synthetic estrogen and progesterone, and a group that they treated with natural supplements.

Both groups had an increase in estrogen levels, but the progesterone levels increased only in the group taking the natural hormones. All the women in the group supplemented with natural estrogen and progesterone reported relief from night sweats and hot flashes within one month. A few of the women in the group taking the synthetic hormonal replacement reported relief from these symptoms, but most did not.

Only the group taking the natural hormonal replacement had significantly lower total cholesterol (Hargrove et. al., 1989).

WHY PHYSICIANS PRESCRIBE SYNTHETIC HORMONES

Reviewing such a study might arouse curiosity about why doctors continue to use synthetic estrogens and progestins in hormonal replacement therapy. Dr. Lee (1993,) believes this occurs for several reasons. One is that many doctors do not know that prescription progestins are made from progesterone that is derived from the Mexican Yam. The pharmaceutical companies alter the molecular form of the substance in order to patent it. A natural substance cannot be patented, which is not profitable, and therefore, the need for the alteration. He also believes that many physicians are unaware that natural progesterone is readily available and is safer and more effective than synthetics, and that natural progesterone is relatively inexpensive. Years ago, yams began being used to produce natural estrogens and progesterones, but pregnant mare's urine is a cheaper and more abundant source and is what is used to manufacture the synthetics by many pharmaceutical companies (Mirkin, 1991). That fact alone is enough to get some reticent women to try natural progesterone. Somehow ingesting an encapsulated powder of yam seems very preferable to ingesting an encapsulated form of pregnant mare's urine.

OSTEOPOROSIS

Osteoporosis is one of the most serious problems of menopause. It can be a crippling, degenerative disease from the progressive loss of bone mass or density, rendering bones thin and brittle, which can lead to skeletal deformities, and leaves its victim at high risk of fractures. This condition occurs when bones are being broken down faster than they are being formed (Werbach, 1993).

Osteoporosis is a disease more common to women. Dr. John Lee in Optimal Health Guidelines states: "Just as coronary heart disease is the disease U.S. men are most certain to develop, so is osteoporosis the disease most U.S. women are certain to develop" (Lee, 1994, p. 89). Gladstar (1993) stated that 25% of American women develop osteoporosis, and the *Doctor's Book of Home Remedies* (1990) states that 24 million Americans have it, with women being the most likely to develop it. Men are not exempt from osteoporosis, but normally develop it later in life when their testosterone levels drop (Lee, Optimal Health, 1993). Only about 8% of men develop the disease in their lifetime (Werbach, 1993).

WHEN DOES OSTEOPOROSIS OCCUR?

Although it is believed that osteoporosis occurs at about the time of menopause in women, this is a misperception according to Dr. John Lee (1993). A female's peak bone mass occurs at about age 30, and a deterioration begins after that. By the time women get to menopause, if they have osteoporosis, it has probably been developing over a number of years.

Bones are constantly renewed or restored in our bodies by the processes called osteoblast and osteoclast. Osteoclast is the process where older and previously mineralized bones are sought out and dissolved. Then the osteoblast moves in and produces new bone. In youth, the osteoblast outperforms the osteoclast, causing us to grow taller and stronger. In adult years, the osteoblast and osteoclast processes keep equal pace. However, after peak bone mass, the osteoblasts begin to slow down, but the osteoclasts keep going, mineralizing more bone than our bodies are renewing, creating the osteoporotic condition (Lee, Optimal Health, 1993).

ABOUT OUR BONES AND OSTEOPOROSIS

There are two kinds of bones in our bodies, cortical and trabecular. The cortical bones are compact, making up 80% of our skeleton. These bones are renewed every ten to fifteen years. The trabecular bones are more spongy and are found in our heel bones, our vertebral bones, and at the ends of long bones. The renewal turnaround time on these bones is every 2-3 years, meaning 40% of them are dissolved and reformed annually (Werbach, 1993). This leaves the trabecular bones much more prone to osteoporosis.

THE RISK OF FRACTURES

The bones where osteoporosis has occurred are very sensitive to fractures. In Optimal Health Guidelines, Dr. Lee (1993) indicates that these bones can become so sensitive that hip fractures can occur with a mere misstep. Perhaps some of the hip fractures blamed on falls actually precede the fall and actually cause the fall.

Osteoporosis is responsible for 1.3 million fractures annually and cost over $10 million in treatment (Lee, 1993). This is medical treatment only and does not take into account the cost many pay in quality and quantity of life due to these fractures. Of these fractures, they occur only in one male for every four fractures in females. Of these fractures, the *Doctors Book of Home Remedies* (1993) quotes Dr. Ken Cooper as saying that 250,000 fractures that occur annually are hip fractures. The seriousness if this is clarified by his report that of those that are 65 years of age or older, 12 to 20% of them die within one year of the fracture.

THE MOST POWERFUL PREVENTION: EXERCISE

This is such a serious disease to aging women, making preventative measures and techniques of prime interest.

Age is not the real culprit of osteoporosis, rather it is a result of poor nutrition, lack of exercise and progesterone deficiency (Lee, 1993). According to Deepak Chopra (1993) in *Ageless Body, Timeless Mind*, the disease is practically unheard of in some tribal societies where physical activity throughout life is the norm. Because we live in a sedentary society, bones get stiff and brittle. Think of it . . . we will drive around a mall parking lot for 15 minutes looking for a close parking space, we will go into a 7-11 and pay a higher price for a loaf of bread than walk to the bakery in the grocery store, and we lose total interest in activities that might require us to stand in line before we take our seat! And remember when there was no remote control and we actually had to get up to change the channel on the television! Escalators and elevators have taken away the opportunity of walking up and down stairs, and golf carts even make a former mild exercise sport less beneficial.

One U.S. study showed that menopausal women who exercise daily for an hour had bone calcium levels increase by a third within a year (Gladstar, 1993). This is ample data to motivate anyone concerned about their health to embark upon a regular exercise program. No longer is exercise just something for thin girls and body-building men, it is a health necessity for those of us wanting to maintain optimal health as we age. If exercise seems like a drudgery to you, join the many "mall walkers" who team up with friends and wall around malls and other indoor public buildings.

ANOTHER GREAT PREVENTION: SEXUAL ACTIVITY

Not all treatments suggested for the prevention and treatment of osteoporosis would seem like such drudgery. According to Dr. Norma McCoy of San Francisco State University and Dr. Julian Davidson of Stanford University, women who continue to participate in sexual intercourse on a regular bases have fewer problems with osteoporosis and hot flashes. (Doctor's Book of Home Remedies, 1990). They believe this is because regular sexual activity moderates the dropping levels of estrogen in the body. Some women (and men) mistakenly believe that menopause is the end of the sexual era for women. How mistaken they both are! This should be a time of enjoyable sexual activity for a couple entering their golden years. It might require some adjustments, such as the use of a lubricant, some hugs and massages to become aroused, but it is definitely not over! Perhaps the topic of sex could instigate some of the heart to heart talks which promote intimacy in these precious years!

OTHER NATURAL TREATMENTS FOR OSTEOPOROSIS

Other natural treatments of osteoporosis may not be as exciting, but are equally beneficial. Most practitioners recognize that calcium and magnesium need to be supplemented. Calcium is recommended to be supplemented at 500 to 600 mg. daily. Calcium rich diets are also recommended: some dairy products, broccoli, collard greens, kale and almonds. Some doctors recommend an increase in milk. However, our bodies need a 1.5 to 2:1 ratio with phosphorous for absorption to take place. The ratio of calcium to phosphorous in a glass of milk is 1:1. Gladstar (1993) points out that the American Dairy Association recommends drinking four glasses of milk daily. We are the only country that promotes such a recommendation and we have the highest rates of osteoporosis. Perhaps you should consider this when attempting to increase your calcium levels with another glass of milk. Horsetail (silica) is often recommended in addition to a calcium rich diet because it aids absorption and utilization of calcium in the body. Magnesium is important because it activates alkaline phosphatase in the system, which is an enzyme that assists in the formation of calcium crystals in the bone.

Vitamin C supplementation of about 500 mg. daily is recommended because of its necessity for activating enzymes needed for collagen synthesis. Collagen is a major component of bone. There are studies that indicate vitamin C deficiency could be a major cause of osteoporosis (Werbach, 1993). Vitamin D is also necessary for the absorption of calcium, but it is recommended that you get it naturally by daily exposure to sunlight.

Another mineral, boron, is a trace element that markedly reduces the excretion of calcium and magnesium in the urine. Both of these are important in the prevention of osteoporosis (Werbach, 1993). Boron elevates the concentration of estradiol in the blood also. You can get it naturally by consuming the following foods: alfalfa, cabbage, lettuce, peas, snap beans, apples, dates, prunes, raisins, almonds, peanuts, and hazel nuts.

Fluorine, or sodium fluoride, is often recommended because it is a potent agent in trabecular bone renewal. However, in the cortical bone mass, it increases fragility. In addition, it can cause damage not the lining of the stomach. Therefore, <u>IT IS NOT RECOMMENDED HERE</u>!

The herbal supplementation recommendations are feverfew and oatstraw. Other mineral supplementation to be considered are copper and phosphorus. The amino acids, L-Lysine and L-Arginine, can be osteoporotic preventatives.

Reduction in the intake of sugar in the form of sucrose and of table salt are highly recommended. Both cause excessive loss of calcium in urine. When the loss of calcium through urine is excessive, post menopausal women are particularly at risk, because the body then causes calcium to be mobilized from its primary place of storage, in the bones, thus promoting osteoporosis. The intake of caffeine promotes the same loss of calcium in both urine and feces, and therefore, should be avoided.

A word of caution should be added here about the consumption of alcohol. Research indicates that alcoholics lose bone density faster than those who do not drink (Werbach, 1993). However, any consumption of alcohol can promote calcium loss, and therefore, bone loss.

NATURAL PROGESTERONE CAN REVERSE OSTEOPOROSIS

What might be the greatest news about natural prevention and treatment of osteoporosis is the use of natural progesterone. To make a candid point, Dr. John Lee (1993) believes that <u>NOT ONLY CAN NATURAL PROGESTERONE SERVE AS A PREVENTION FOR OSTEOPOROSIS, BUT IT CAN ACTUALLY REVERSE OSTEOPOROSIS</u>.

As seen in the chart below, postmenopausal women with osteoporosis lose about 1.5% of their bone mass annually, Those on estrogen supplements seem to be able to maintain their loss. However, those on natural progesterone actually show an increase in their bone mineral density. Dr. Lee in

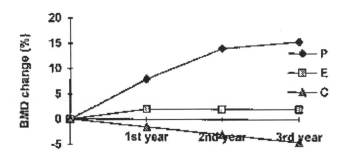

Typical lumbar BMD changes with
progesterone (P), estrogen only (E), or
control (C)

Optimal Health Guidelines (1993) stated that "only the addition of progesterone will increase bone mass, thus reversing the osteoporotic process" (p. 95).

Dr. Lee conducted a study in 1990 with 100 postmenopausal women. Each woman was placed on a special diet, emphasizing leafy green vegetables, limiting red meat and alcohol, eliminating all carbonated beverages. Vitamin D was supplemented at 350-400 i.u. daily and Vitamin C was administered in 2,000 mg. daily. Calcium was ingested at 800-1000 mg/day through diet and/or supplements. Conjugated oestrogen was given three weeks out of the month, and natural progesterone was given transdermally daily for twelve days of the month. Patients on this regimen were followed for at least three years. Treatment results were broad and very positive, including: stabilization of height, diminished aches and pains, rise in energy levels, return of normal libido, no rise in lipid levels, and no adverse side effects. Bone density studies done every six months to one year show a progressive increase in bone mass. The first six to twelve months showed a 3 to 5% increase until stabilizing at the levels of a healthy 35 year old woman. The increases were faster in those who had lower bone densities in the beginning. The occurrence of osteoporotic fractures dropped to zero. Three women during the study had bone fractures in accidents unrelated to osteoporosis. Not only did they experience complete healing, but their treating orthopedic physicians commented on the excellent healing and bone structure for women their age. There were no complaints of gastric irritations, stiffness, headaches or moodiness. Dr. Lee (1990) summarizes the study by stating: "The results shown in this study suggest that osteoporosis is not an irreversible condition. Reversal has been demonstrated by the bone density tests and by the clinical results. This can not be said of any other conventional therapy for osteoporosis" (p. 389). He added that the use of natural progesterone is obviously safe, uncomplicated, and inexpensive.

WHY NATURAL PROGESTERONE IS SO EFFECTIVE

The reason the natural progesterone is so important in the treatment of osteoporosis is its effect on the osteoblast renewal mentioned earlier in this chapter. Progesterone stimulates the osteoblastic renewal process in bones, which results in new bone formation. Therefore, the lack of progesterone can cause osteoporosis by the lack of new bone formation. Dr. Lee (1993) states: "Postmenopausal osteoporosis is a disease of inadequate osteoblast-mediated new bone formation secondary to progesterone deficiency. Progesterone restores osteoblast function. Natural progesterone hormone is an essential factor in the prevention and proper treatment of osteoporosis" (p. 69).

As you can see in the Biochemical Pathway chart in Appendix A. DHEA is a prehormone which has no biologic potency in and of itself. It can be converted to estrone or estradiol from natural supplements derived from the Mexican Yam (Leiter et. al., 1987, p. 863). This indicates that DHEA could provide a steroidal postmenopausal replacement that is to estrogens (Buster et.al., 1992).

Dr. John Lee (1993) addresses the issue of using estrogen replacement therapy with natural progesterone. He first points out that estrogen levels do not drop to zero with menopause because she continues to make it through androstenedione in fat cells. However, if it falls below what she needs, natural hormones derived from the Mexican Yam can easily be converted to those estrogens as easily as it can be to progesterones through pregnenolone (See Biochemical Pathway in Appendix).

THE GOOD NEWS

To summarize the great news in this chapter, you don't have to suffer from the discomforting symptoms of menopause and osteoporosis. The keys are: get up, get active, take natural products derived from the Mexican Yam, eat (healthily – leafy green veggies, in particular), drink (but not carbonated beverages or alcohol), and be merry (with all the sexual activity you like).

6

PREMENSTRUAL SYNDROME: THE BATTLE OF THE HORMONES AND THE EFFECTS OF DHEA

Until recent years, premenstrual syndrome, PMS, was primarily considered a malady that existed only in the "head" or "emotions" of women. However, as far back as 50 years ago, research was being conducted to determine the causes of and treatments for PMS (Frank, 1931). Knowing that research has been going on that long makes it very difficult to believe that PMS remains so unacknowledged and so misunderstood. Not only has the research been in progress for many years, but the numbers of women suffering from this condition are astounding. According to the PMS Self-Help Center in Los Altos, California, more than half the women in the U. S. suffer from PMS monthly.

Women, since the beginning of recorded history, have consistently reported the discomforts and symptoms of PMS, yet it continued to remain unrecognized. Perhaps it may seem sexist to say so, but much of the literature points to the possibility that the complaints may have been ignored because male doctors were unable to understand the complaints, or were unsympathetic because of no ability to relate to the monthly symptoms being described. This sentiment is expressed pointedly in *Herbal Healing for Women*: "Until recently, PMS was regarded by the medical community primarily as an imaginary dis-ease. I wonder if men were to suffer monthly from severe debilitating cramps, joint pain, bloating, headaches, and excess bleeding if PMS would be so easily dismissed as imaginary or "all in the head" (Gladstar, 1993, pp. 124-125). One doctor was quoted as stating that women should not be considered for leadership positions due to the emotional imbalances of PMS, which he called "raging hormonal influences" (Kamen, 1993, p. 48).

And it has not been due to the complaints of women suffering that the medical profession has finally turned its attention to PMS; rather, it has been the result of PMS being used as a legal defense by lawyers that has turned the medical community's attention to the realities of PMS. In the early 1980's, the British court system reduced murder charges to manslaughter in the cases of two women because they were thought to have had "diminished responsibility" as a result of their PMS (Lauersen and Stukane, 1983). In three different murder trials in Great Britain, the women were "sentenced" to take progesterone to treat their PMS, which was supposedly the cause of them committing violent crimes.

THE AWFUL SYMPTOMS OF PMS

PMS is a conglomeration of symptoms that occurs monthly anywhere from two to ten days before menstruation and can continue until menstruation begins or even a few days following the onset. The symptom conglomeration includes such complaints as: cramping, bloating, abdominal swelling, headaches, excessive menstrual flow, constipation, nervousness, frequent urination, cravings for salts and sweets, breast tenderness, sleep disturbance, clumsiness, loss of libido, acne, moodiness, irritability, water retention, fatigue, and depression. These symptoms can range from mild to severe. When symptoms become extremely severe, other symptoms may accompany these, such as: agitation, cyclic depressions, asthma attacks, seizures, migraine headaches, loss of motor coordination, emotional instability, and suicidal ideation (Lauersen and Stukane, 1983).

THE CAUSES OF PMS

Writers, doctors and researchers have stated a variety of reasons for the cause of PMS. Dr. Abraham (1986) pointed to hormonal imbalances; Gladstar (1993) indicated negative images of menstruation, childhood abuse, and hormonal imbalance; Drs. Stieglitz and Kimble (1949) reported the cause as a toxic condition in the body; Dr. Rose (1978) found the cause to be a Vitamin B deficiency; Dr. Lee (1994) stated the cause to be "anovulatory cycles in sensitive women whose emotional and physiological balance is upset by stress and/or improper diet" (p. 12); Dr. Kamen (1993) added factors such as: thyroid hypofunction, antidiuretic hormone excess, serotonin alterations, and yeast overgrowth. Whatever the cause, PMS is finally becoming recognized as a "real" condition, even by the medical community.

THE BATTLE OF THE HORMONES

Although there may be a lack of clarity about the exact role hormones play in PMS, most doctors and researchers agree that a hormonal imbalance of some sort is at the very least a contributor to, if not the cause of, PMS. The *Doctor's Book of Home Remedies* (1990) portrays the imbalance as a war within a woman's body. "Think of it as biological warfare, its battles played out on the fields of a woman's body and mind. Once a month, about two weeks before her menstrual period, the opposing armies – estrogen and progesterone – begin to amass. These female hormones, which regulate her menstrual cycle and affect her central nervous system, normally work in tandem. It's only when one tries to outdo the other that trouble looms.

Some women escape the conflict altogether; their hormones strike a peaceful balance before a single sword is drawn. Others are less fortunate. For one woman, estrogen levels may soar; leaving her feeling anxious and irritable. Or her progesterone predominates, dragging her into depression and fatigue. The battles can rage on for days. And then, suddenly, the troops clear out and peace of mind returns . . . " (p. 505).

So the battle of PMS is actually primarily between estrogen on one side and progesterone on the other. Both are produced in both the ovaries and the adrenals (Cutler, 1988). The normal variation for these hormones is shown in the chart below.

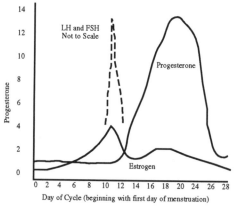

Day of Cycle (beginning with first day of menstruation)

As pictured, the progesterone levels begin to rise at the time of ovulation and continue to remain peaked until menstruation. However, in PMS sufferers, the progesterone levels are significantly lower during those two weeks between ovulation and the onset of menstruation (Kamen, 1988). It is unclear exactly why the progesterone levels are lower in women who suffer with PMS. Perhaps the ovaries are not producing enough, or the hypothalamus and pituitary glands are not producing as they should, or stress levels are effecting its production.

Regardless of why the hormonal imbalance exists, it is clear that there are physiological realities that a woman experiences due to these imbalances. It is clear that as progesterone levels rise, it has a seemingly narcotic effect, a "pleasant sleepiness" (Cutler, 1988, p. 16). As progesterone levels fall, depression occurs. When the estrogen and progesterone levels are balanced properly, an emotional harmony ensues.

Dr. Abraham (1986) conducted a study and described how hormones and symptoms interact during PMS. He noted premenstrual anxiety to be characterized by an elevation in estrogen and low levels of progesterone. He attributed premenstrual depression to elevated progesterone levels later in the cycle, along with an increase in the male hormones, the androgens. He described premenstrual cravings to be characterized by evidence of reactive hypoglycemia. He associated fluid retention with elevated aldosterone, a male hormone. Although many studies have been performed to understand the impact of various hormones on the PMS cycle, there is a paucity of research in the area of the role of androgens in PMS (Eriksson et. al., 1992, p. 196).

THE NORMAL RISE AND FALL OF HORMONES

According to Dr. John Lee (1993), the normal rise and fall of hormones through a female's monthly cycle is as follows: The first week following menses is characterized by estrogen dominance; during ovulation, progesterone levels begin to increase until they are dominant two weeks preceding menstruation. He cites that the real problem begins when there is a surplus of estrogen or a progesterone deficiency in these two weeks. Then he believes that a deficiency of progesterone effects the regulatory hypothalamic centers, causing them to become hyperactive. He also believes that the progesterone deficiency can increase production of FSH (follicule

stimulating hormone) and LH (luteinizing hormone) gona-
dotropins, which play a role in PMS. However, he has found
that simply supplementing his patients with natural progesterone cream restores the hormonal feedback system and that
the pituitary function becomes normal once again. If the PSH
and LH levels are elevated two to ten days preceding menstruation, it indicates that the estrogen and progesterone levels are imbalanced.

HAVING YOUR HORMONES CHECKED

Blood analyses can be done to determine a woman's hormonal balances, yet it is amazing how many doctors, including gynecologists, do not conduct this test or order it , even in
women who have premenstrual complaints. Lauersen and
Stukane (1983) suggest that five different hormones should
be checked when a female is being screened for PMS: 1)
Check the level of the hormone prolactin. Prolactin, one of
the pituitary hormones, causes the production of breast milk.
It is often elevated in PMS. 2) Check is the thyroid hormones. The thyroid stimulates the brain to release FSH and
LH, which cause the menstrual cycle to begin. When these
are deficient, it could hinder the production of progesterone,
leading to PMS symptoms. 3) Check the FSH and LH hormonal levels. The brain communicates hormonally with the
pituitary gland and to begin menstruation. The pituitary re-
leases FSH into the blood, which travels to the ovaries. In
the ovaries, the FSH stimulates the production of estrogen.
The pituitary then notes the increase in estrogen and sends
out LH to stop the FSH. This causes ovulation to begin, which
only lasts about 24 hours. High levels of LH and FSH during
the premenstrual days is a sign of hormonal imbalance. 4)
The female hormones, estradiol and progesterone are direct
clues to PMS hormonal imbalances. The important key in

checking these hormones is their ratio one to another, and the phase of the cycle during which the test is conducted. If these ratios are imbalanced, PMS could be indicated. 5) Check the levels of the male hormone testosterone.

TREATING PMS:
PRESCRIPTION DRUGS OR NATURAL PRODUCTS

Just as there are a variety of ideas regarding the cause of PMS, there are also a variety of ideas about treating PMS. In the past, women have been treated as if they were mentally ill when reporting the symptoms of PMS and were given tranquilizers or other inappropriate medications. As stated by Dr. Corsello (1994, p. 3): "Women suffer mood swings. [But] this only defines one manifestation of the problem and continues to stigmatize its victims by labeling it with psychological or emotionally-based symptoms. This is no doubt that PMS is accompanied by a great deal of emotional turmoil, but that is not the cause of the problem – it is the effect."

With the medical profession finally realizing that there is more to PMS than mood swings, new treatment ideas have emerged. Treatments include everything from hormonal supplementation, nutritional changes, stress reduction, environmental adaptations, lifestyle changes, exercise regimens, and vitamin supplementation.

Natural herbal treatments have provided relief for some sufferers of PMS. Studies conducted in London and Canada indicated that women with severe PMS were treated successfully with evening primrose oil, and following treatment reported an incredible reduction the symptoms of irritability, headaches, breast tenderness, and bloating (Mindell, 1992). Dong quai, another herbal remedy has been shown to eliminate the discomforts of PMS. Borage, another natural substance, contains gamma lineoleic acid, a substance which has been known to successfully treat PMS.

Vitamin supplementation is another regimen used to treat PMS. Lauersen and Stukane (1983) recommend 800 to 1,000 mgs of Vitamin E daily, 400 mg of vitamin D, 2 to 3 grams of calcium, Vitamin B-complex 300 to 800 mg (with extra Vitamin B6), 50 mg of zinc, and 1000 mg of Vitamin C (p. 56). *The Doctor's Book of Home Remedies* recommends vitamin supplementation as well. Vitamin B6 is recommended because of research indicates it can alleviate mood swings, fluid retention, breast tenderness, bloating, sugar cravings, and fatigue. Vitamin A and D are recommended to suppress the possibilities of or outbreaks of premenstrual acne or other skin problems. Vitamin C is recommended because of its antioxidant effect of reducing stress. Vitamin E also has the antioxidant effect, and is believed to relieve breast tenderness, anxiety and depression. Calcium and magnesium can work together to relieve cramps, subside cravings, and stabilize the mood swings common to PMS. L-tyrosine, an amino acid, can serve as a natural antidepressant.

Diet is another area to assess in addressing the symptoms of PMS. Kamen (1993) reported that physicians and women both found PMS symptoms disappeared when they switched to a nutrient-dense diet. Mindell (1992) recommended the following dietary changes: avoiding salty foods, eating herbs that have natural diuretic properties (alfalfa, asparagus, celery, dandelion, carrots), avoiding caffeine, and drinking chamomile tea.

EXERCISE AND PMS

Exercise is another highly recommended way to alleviate the symptoms of PMS. Women in good physical condition are less likely to experience the symptoms and discomforts of PMS (Lauersen and Stukane, 1983). Cutler (1988) recommends regular exercise because it increases endorphin levels and increases blood circulation. She also noted that women only need to work at 60% of their maximum capacity to achieve these results. One of the mistakes PMS sufferers can make is to begin an exercise program with too much exertion too quickly, resulting in exhaustion or injury, followed by returning to a sedentary lifestyle. A consistent, gradually built exercise program is recommended.

Exercise also contributes to improved levels of beta endorphins. This is an important factor to consider because research indicates that PMS sufferers have a reduction in beta endorphin levels during the days they suffer from the symptoms of PMS, and their beta endorphin levels peak up to five times greater than other women's levels at the time of ovulation (Cutler, 1988). This incredible rise and severe decline of beta endorphins in women suffering from PMS is one of the reasons for the depressed mood that accompanies other symptoms. Truly, the depression is not just a "woman's thing", but it is obviously a true chemical imbalance in the woman's body, which is beyond her control. However, some practical things, such as exercise, can moderate those chemical imbalances and bring some relief.

OTHER PRACTICAL REMEDIES

There are a variety of other practical remedies recommended that anyone suffering from PMS could employ. For example, several small meals daily as opposed to large meals can make the chemical imbalances less radical. It is suggested that no junk foods, particularly those full of sugar, be eaten. Dairy products should be limited because the lactose in dairy products can block the body's ability to absorb magnesium which can help to regulate estrogen levels in the body. Other dietary tips include: lowering the intake of sodium, increasing the intake of fiber, avoiding caffeine and alcohol. Learning to pamper yourself can also go a long way in relieving some of the symptoms: De-stress your environment, treat yourself to mineral baths and massages, don't push yourself into social events you don't feel up to, stick to a relaxed schedule, catch up on your sleep prior to your PMS days when you know you won't sleep well. "Hormones, especially those in the brain, are extremely sensitive to a woman's daily regimens – diet, exercise, sleep patterns – and these hormones can rise or fall if a woman suddenly allows a routine activity either to become excessive or to vanish" (Lauersen and Stukane, 1983, p. 57).

Estrogen/progesterone levels are also shown to be regulated when a regimen of regular sexual activity is followed by PMS sufferers (Cutler, 1988). Perhaps this is because those who participate in regular sexual activity are more fertile. This is important because even if a woman is not desiring pregnancy, higher fertility reflects higher levels of health in the endocrine system.

PSYCHOTHERAPY AND PMS

Individual, marital, and family therapy have been indicated in the course of treatment for some individuals suffering with PMS. Dr. Guy Abraham, in *The Doctor's Book of Home Remedies* stated PMS as a major cause of divorce. Many husbands do not understand the dynamics of the changes that occur in their wives bodies monthly. Unfortunately, many wives do not understand it themselves and find themselves frustrated in their futile attempts to explain their symptoms, their behaviors, and their moods. Although psychotherapy may not be curative in and of itself, educational therapy can certainly be helpful in assisting couples understand, cope with, and improve the symptoms of PMS. In support of the therapeutic process as a tool in treatment, Lauersen and Stukane state: "A woman's husband, family, and friends might be more crucial than any medical specialist in helping her to overcome PMS. [Therefore] often families need counseling as much as women themselves. Now that he and she both realize that PMS is the problem, he must call upon his patience, sensitivity, and understanding to make the home environment as serene as possible, to reduce the stress and the guilt that can often intensify symptoms" (1983, p. 113). One of the most helpful aspects of therapy is to demystify the notion that PMS is a form of "insanity." Currently, the Diagnostic and Statistics Manual of Mental Disorders lists PMS as a mental disorder, not otherwise specified. This kind of documentation supports the idea that PMS is a mental condition, which it clearly is NOT! Good therapy can help the women suffering with PMS, her husband, and her family understand the physiological realities of the condition, as well as help all involved work together to deal with the condition.

NATURAL PROGESTERONE AND PMS

All of the above listed treatments have some effect on the symptoms of PMS, however, Dr. John Lee believes that all of these helpful things exclude one of the most beneficial treatments available to women suffering from PMS: the use of natural progesterone. When he began prescribing natural progesterone in the treatment of women suffering from PMS, he found "the majority (but not all) of such patients reported remarkable improvement in the symptom-complex, including the elimination of their premenstrual water retention and weight gain" (1993, p. 50).

As mentioned earlier, it is unclear exactly why progesterone deficiencies occur after ovulation in women who experience PMS. But many practitioners report successful results according to their observation and according to the reports given by their patients when natural progesterone treatment is employed. Dr. Kamen states that "there is evidence that natural progesterone supplementation works to alleviate PMS in the majority of cases" (1993, p.213). She also includes statements made by other doctors. Dr. Kirk noted that her patients refer to natural progesterone as miraculous. Dr. Marx found no other substance more effective than natural progesterone to relieve the symptoms of PMS. Dr. Corsello noted that young women found natural progesterone supplementation made a tremendous difference. Dr. Kunin observed his patients finding relief in less than 15 minutes when supplemented with natural progesterone. Dr. Lee reported patients experiencing a remarkable change in the quality of their lives when supplemented with natural progesterone (Kamen, 1993, pp. 210-211). Dr. Joel T. Hargrove published an article in *McCalls* Magazine in 1990 where he stated that he had achieved a 90% success rate when treating women orally suffering from PMS with natural progesterone. Dr. Lauersen exclaimed: "PMS is real and progesterone helps to cure it if a hormonal imbalance is found" (Lauersen and Stukane, 1983, p. 172).

Dr. Kamen (1993, p. 14) states the benefit of natural progesterone very clearly: "There is impressive evidence that natural progesterone can correct a critical deficiency that may prove to be the real cause of PMS." Dr. John Lee clearly supports this statement by one of his own: "Appropriate treatment requires correction of this hormone imbalance and the most effective technique, at present, for achieving this is supplemental natural progesterone" (Lee, 1993, p. 52). The emphasis here is on natural progesterone. Research indicates that synthetic progesterone can inhibit the concentration of natural progesterone, which can further upset the imbalance of hormones, causing an intensification of PMS symptoms (Kamen, 1992, p. 213). *The Physician's Desk Reference* (1994) lists the side effects of one of the synthetic progesterones (medroxyprogesterone acetate): possible adverse effects on fetus, breast tenderness, edema, acne, breakthrough bleeding, spotting, changes in weight, jaundice, depression, insomnia, nausea. When taken in conjunction with synthetic estrogen, the following side effects were listed: premenstrual-like syndrome, changes in libido (sexual desire), changes in appetite, headache, nervousness, fatigue, loss of scalp hair, itching. One would have to ask why a synthetic progesterone would be used when multiples of researchers have concluded that natural progesterone is more beneficial and has less side effects than synthetic progestins (Fahraeus et al, 1983, p. 447). Kamen quotes a conversation with Dr. John Lee, in which he stated, "There are no known side effects from natural progesterone, which, as should be obvious to all, is the preferred from to use if supplementation is to be given" (Kamen, 1993, p. 207).

This natural form of progesterone can be supplemented to the body through the natural use of herbal products derived from Dioscorea Villosa. Women taking this form of natural oral supplementation report incredible results.

"IT'S LIKE A MIRACLE"

A good friend and colleague of mine, whom I will call Elizabeth, learned about the natural precursor products about five months ago. As an open-minded health care provider, she began taking the supplements. By two months after she had started taking the supplements, she noticed her PMS symptoms were not quite as bad. She didn't make the connection between the supplements and the PMS at all, until her husband brought home an article he had seen featured in *Natural Health* in March/April entitled: "Treating PMS Without Side Effects".

About seven years ago, at age 34, Elizabeth experienced awful symptoms two weeks before her period. She had terrible depression, her breasts become swollen and extremely tender. She would experience a five pound weight gain from water retention, and feel bloated. She would experience a 5 to 10 times increase in appetite, craving sweets. She said she would eat, and eat, and despite feeling physically full, she felt she could never get enough to eat. She also felt incredibly irritable during these two weeks and although she could function appropriately at work, she really didn't feel like doing anything social.

She had seen a doctor who gave her prozac and diuretics. They helped some, but she didn't want to stay on those medications. Now, just five months after she began taking the natural progesterone made from the Mexican Yam, she states: Iit's like a miracle." She is free of PMS symptoms and her prescription medications taken to treat them.

7

DHEA: CAN IT LOWER CHOLESTEROL?

All that many of us know about cholesterol is that there are many products on the supermarket shelf now that have bold letters advertising that they are "cholesterol free" or "low in cholesterol." We know we need to watch our cholesterol and keep it down, but that may be the sum total of our understanding about what it does, where it comes from, and how to keep it at healthy levels.

CHOLESTEROL ≠ FAT

One of the greatest misunderstandings I find among the people I work and consult with is the false correlation between fat and cholesterol. Cholesterol and fat are not the same when noted on food labeling. You might choose something that is "cholesterol free," yet it might be loaded with fat.

THE GOOD GUYS AND THE BAD GUYS OF CHOLESTEROL

A quick biological explanation may help clarify what cholesterol is and what purpose it serves in our bodies. Lipopro-

teins are the vehicles in our blood which transport cholesterol. LDL (low density lipoproteins) carry about 65% of
our cholesterol throughout our system. LDL are the guys
with the "black hats." They leave deposits of cholesterol in
the arteries that can cause plaque build up, and then block
our arteries.

Our VLDL (very low density lipoproteins) carry only
about 15% of our cholesterol through our system, but they
are the guys with "really black hats". They not only can leave
the same deposits, but they are what the liver needs to make
more LDL. So the "really bad guys" (VLDL) promote the
production of the "bad guys" (LDL) which can increase risk
of coronary disease (Mindell, 1991).

As in every good Western, there are "good guys" in this
scenario. The "good guys" are HDL (high density lipoproteins) and they carry about 20% of the cholesterol throughout our system. These "good guys" are "really good guys"
because they are composed of lechitin. Lechitin performs a
scrubbing action in the arteries, breaking up and clearing out
plaque build up left behind by the "bad guys" (LDL).

Biochemically speaking, cholesterol is an organic compound with the structure of a fatty alcohol. Not only is cholesterol not bad for us, but it is necessary for some major
bodily functions. It converts sunlight to Vitamin D when its
ultraviolet rays touch the skin. It aids in the metabolism of
carbohydrates. It is a prime supplier of adrenal steroid hormones, and is necessary for production of male and female
sex hormones. It is a component of every membrane in our
bodies, and is used to build protective membranes in our cells.
These membranes prevent substances from entering or leaving our cells. It also is a protective skin barrier. It is because
of cholesterol that we lose only ten to 14 ounces of water
daily through evaporation.

Triglycerides are related types of blood fats that travel

with cholesterols in the blood as lipoproteins. Higher levels of triglycerides can cause blood cells to stick together and impair circulation, ending in heart attacks or strokes. The major connection between triglycerides and cholesterol that is pertinent to our subject is that lowering triglycerides also helps lower cholesterol (Mindell, 1991, p. 125).

IDEAL LEVELS OF HDL AND LDL

So what are the ideal levels of the "good guy" and "bad guy" cholesterols and what difference does it make? Up until recently, if your cholesterol was checked, you were given one number. Now it is very important to know your HDL level (the level of the "good guys") and the LDL level (the level of the "bad guys").

Recently, I was teaching some children about cholesterol and how important it was. I was saying that they could remember that LDL were the "bad guys" by imagining that the LDL stood for "low down life." I said I hadn't yet thought of what "HDL" could stand for to represent the "good guys." A teacher quickly informed me that HDL could stand for the "Howdy Doodey Life." However you remember it, it is important to remember that we want less of the "bad guys" (LDL) and more of the "good guys" (HDL). Ideally, the LDL level needs to stay knocked down below 200, and the HDL rates need to stay elevated above 35, according to a recent article in Consumer Reports on Health (1994, p. 28).

The same report revealed a study conducted in Europe over a five year period studying over 4,000 men. It was noted that raising their HDL levels 11% and lowering their LDL levels 11% cut their risk of heart disease by one-third (1994, p. 28). They reported another study conducted by the John Hopkins University that followed 1400 older women for 14 years. They noted that in these women, high LDL levels did not seem to increase their risk for death due to coronary disease. However, those women who had low, or even moderately low, HDL levels had an increased risk of 200% of dying of coronary disease (1994, p. 29).

SYMPTOMS OF HIGH LDL AND LOW HDL CHOLESTEROL

High LDL cholesterol levels are the primary cause of heart disease. In addition, those high levels can also lead to clogging of the arteries, gall stones, high blood pressure, impotence, and mental impairment (Nyholt, 1993, p. 44). The symptoms of high LDL and low HDL levels are varied and diverse. They can include some things you might notice, such as: leg cramps and pain, difficulty breathing, cold hands and feet, dry skin and hair, lethargy, dizziness, allergies; or they can include symptoms you might not readily notice, such as: plaque forming on the artery walls, poor circulation, high blood pressure, palpitations, kidney problems.

There is debate about dietary alterations and their effect on cholesterol levels. Dr. Morter (1993, p, 171) claims that a moderate reduction in intake of cholesterol can alter your levels by 15% and that extreme changes in dietary consumption of cholesterol can result in up to a 30% improvement in cholesterol levels. Others disagree. Dr. Gordon, in the well-known Farmington study noted that there was little or no correlation between dietary change and cholesterol levels (Amazing Medicines the Drug Companies Don't Want You to Discover!, 1993, p. 204). Even those who decide to monitor food intake to reduce LDL cholesterol levels get mixed advice. Some sources recommend removing all eggs from the diet. However, egg consumption is now half of what it was in 1945 in the U.S., yet there is no comparable reduction in heart disease. Others not only say that eating eggs should not be stopped, but that it might also raise HDL levels (Mindell, 1991, p. 124). Those are the "good guys" whose levels we want to see elevated.

NATURAL TREATMENTS FOR HIGH CHOLESTEROL

Mindell (1991, pp. 125-126) has listed some nutrients and food that he believes will lower LDL cholesterol levels. The list includes activated charcoal, barley, carrots, chromium, corn bran, broccoli, cauliflower, eggplant, evening primrose oil, funugreek seed, fiber, EPA and DHA fish oils, garlic, ginger, guar gum, lemon grass, pinto, lima, navy and kidney beans, olive, peanut and canola oil, niacin, oat bran, onions, apples, grapefruit, beta sitosterol, psyllium husk, red pepper, rice bran, soy beans, Vitamins C and E, and yogurt. He warned to discontinue the following to lower LDL levels: smoking, intake of caffeine, exposure to stress, use of the pill for birth control, intake of refined sugar and food additives, exposure to environmental pollutants (Mindell, 1991, p. 126).

The Doctor's Book of Home Remedies (1990) recommends watching weight as the most important factor in cholesterol reduction. They reported a twenty year study in the Netherlands where body weight was found to be the most important determinant of serum cholesterol. In Airola's *Worldwide Secrets for Staying Young* (1982), he revealed one study that showed ginseng to reduce the amount of cholesterol accumulated in the arteries, and dramatically improve circulation (p. 110). He also hailed garlic as an important nutrient to treat high LDL cholesterol levels.

NATURAL TREATMENT TO RAISE HDL LEVELS

It is important to also note ways to elevate the HDL levels. A regular aerobic exercise program is definitely the best way to raise those levels without medication. One research project noted that inactive people had HDL levels under 40, while joggers had levels over 60, and marathon runners had levels exceeding 70. This study is very important in prevention of and in treatment of HDL levels. It is important to note that aerobic exercise does not lower LDL levels. However, strength training, or non aerobic types of exercise lower LDL levels, but do not raise HDL levels. This provides the answer to the questions of "do I need an aerobic exercise program" or a "strength training program"? The answer is that we need BOTH!

RESEARCH ABOUT DHEA AND CHOLESTEROL

Once again, we can turn to the use of DHEA, or its natural precursor, for the treatment of cholesterol levels. In one study, doctors at the Medical College of Virginia administered daily doses of DHEA. The results were a 7% reduction in the LDL cholesterol levels. And it might be interesting to note that the subjects in this test did not have high LDL levels in the first place. ("Medical News", 1988). Another interesting study involved New Zealand white rabbits who were supplemented with DHEA and who were fed a high cholesterol diet. Results indicated that there was a 30 to 40% inhibition of buildup in the veins (Arad, et. Al., 1989).

A study with rhesus monkeys was conducted to determine whether or not DHEA would lower serum cholesterol levels. Using twelve monkeys, half received DHEA, and half received placebos daily for two months. The LDL cholesterol levels were markedly decreased in the monkeys receiving the DHEA. There was no significant increase in HDL levels, however, there were several monkeys on the DHEA who had slight increases in HDL levels. This study is important because it is believed that the endocrine system of the monkey is very similar to that of humans (Mac Ewen, et.al., 1990).

Diosgenin, the precursor complex derived from the Mexican Yam, Dioscorea Villosa, has also been studied regarding its ability to reduce cholesterol. Studies have found that it does lower blood and liver cholesterol levels (Zagoya, J.C.D., et. al., 1971). In a study done with monkeys, it was found that diosgenin (as well as some other saponins) prevented high cholesterol levels even when they were fed high cholesterol diets (Malinow, 1985).

ONE WOMAN'S SUCCESS STORY

Recently, one of my colleagues began taking a natural precursor complex tablet in hopes to lose some weight. Her major concern was how it would effect her already elevated LDL levels. I assured her that research indicated that her levels could be affected all right, but in a positive way, lowering them. She was hesitant, but consulted with her physician on my advice, and decided to give it a thirty day trial. She brought by a copy of her blood work done one month after starting her supplements (and I had a copy of her blood work from the month before she began taking them). Her LDL level was 214 before beginning the supplement, but her new result sheet sporting a score of 169, sporting a bright red circle drawn around it by her physician with the words: "Excellent improvement" scrawled out beside it!

8

DHEA'S EFFECT ON ARTHRITIS
AND MULTIPLE SCLEROSIS

ARTHRITIS

Arthritis may be one of the oldest conditions known on earth since it has been discovered that cave men and dinosaurs had it. Nearly 40 million Americans have rheumatoid arthritis, and another 16 million have osteoarthritis (Null,1992). Rheumatoid arthritis, the most common type, is normally described as morning stiffness that seems to improve as the day goes on. Rheumatoid arthritis, a systemic disease, is characterized by chronic swelling of joints, muscles, ligaments and tendons.

Exact etiology of the disease is unclear, but there are a number of probable causes: insufficient calcium, lack of hormones, glandular imbalances, poor diets, prolonged use of aspirin, long-term use of steroid drugs (prednisone, etc.), osteoporosis, auto-toxemia from constipation. Because the cause of both of these can be osteoporosis, hormonal imbalance, once again it is helpful to look at the research available regarding DHEA and this condition. Since the treatment of arthritis costs Americans more than $13 billion annually, it is time to take a serious look at alternative, safe treatments, preferably natural treatments (Null, 1992).

DHEA TREATMENT OF ARTHRITIS

One study conducted in London involved 185 postmenopausal women, aged 45-65, who were diagnosed with rheumatoid arthritis. It found that those who were not on any steroid treatment of any kind had low DHEA levels. Those who were on prescription steroid treatments had even lower levels. Even those who had previously been on prescription steroids had lower DHEA levels than those who had not previously been on steroid therapy. (This suggests that there is a recovery period for the adrenals, even after prescription steroid treatment has been ceased). The reasons for the lowered levels of DHEA in rheumatoid arthritis remain unclear, but could be due to chronic illness (shown to reduce DHEA levels), immune dysfunction, or a defect of the adrenal system (Hall et.al., 1993).

In the chapter regarding hormonal replacement therapy and osteoporosis, it was well validated how those conditions could be treated with a natural precursor complex from the Mexican Yam, which can convert through pregnenolone to DHEA or progesterone in our bodies. Dr. Ward Dean (1993) states that "despite the lack of human experience with pregnenolone, . . . it is well known historically as a treatment for arthritis" (p. 81). Perhaps the natural products derived from the Mexican Yam can provide safe, nontoxic relief for sufferers of arthritis.

MULTIPLE SCLEROSIS

Multiple sclerosis is a chronic disease of the central nervous system, thought to be triggered by allergens. The disease is the result of damage to the sheaths of nerve cells in the brain and spinal cord. It has been deemed an incurable disease because the immune system fights against itself. The common symptoms include numbness, severe fatigue, weakness, visual disturbances and/or loss, difficulty breathing, slurring of the speech, poor motor coordination, tremors, dizziness, and nerve degeneration. There are many theories about what causes multiple sclerosis, including a diet comprised of excess carbohydrates and saturated fats, lead or heavy metal poisoning, hypoglycemia, deficiencies of Vitamins B6, B12, or B1, gland imbalance, and food allergies which trigger an auto-immune reaction. One theory suggests viral or bacterial infection as the initiator of the auto-immune reaction.

More women than men seem to be afflicted with this disease, with the age of onset commonly being between 25 and 40. The disease seems to operate in one of two different ways. One way is a cycle of remission and relapse, the other is chronically progressive. Spontaneous remission is rare. If a person with M.S. experiences stabilization or improvement at all, it is considered a significant outcome.

USE OF DHEA IN TREATING MULTIPLE SCLEROSIS

Several recent studied suggest that DHEA and DHEA-S may be effective in the fight against multiple sclerosis. DHEA plays an important role in cellular control, immunoregulation and in the maintenance of the metabolic and structural integrity of the nervous tissue. There is also some evidence that DHEA may have antiviral properties. When summed up, these studies indicated that DHEA's role may be in rebalancing the complex malfunctioning of the immune, neural, and metabolic systems so often seen in M.S.

One study (Roberts et.al., 1990) observed 21 patients, nine males and 12 females, all in the chronic state of M.S. DHEA was administered orally for several months to these patients. Previous to the study, all but one of the patients had lower than normal levels of DHEA. Blood levels of DHEA and DHEA-S increased to normal or above normal after the administration of the DHEA. Data was then gathered from patient-physician interviews and from interviews with the caregivers of the patients. There was discernible improvement in the daily quality of life in three of the nine females and seven of the 12 male patients. The females reported increased energy levels, greater limb strength, better dexterity, and more power in the lower limbs. One patient also reported an increase in libido. Two of the three patients who reported these results noted that when the DHEA treatment stopped, so did the improvements they had noted. The male patients reported increased energy levels and endurance, fewer episodes of incontinence, and a decreased sense of numbness. Four of the seven also noted significant changes for the better in their sexual performance. All reported substantial reductions in improvements when the DHEA was stopped.

Another study using DHEA with M.S. patients noted that 64% of the patients felt relief from the fatigue so often associated with M.S. This has implications for those suffering from chronic fatigue as well (Calabrese, et.al, 1990).

The results of these studies are quite encouraging in an otherwise dismal field, as far as treatments offered for a chronic disease. The recognition by researchers that DHEA may play an important role in such a complex disease, is quite significant. Perhaps the supplements derived from the Mexican Wild Yam would provide hope for M.S. patients.

9

DHEA : AN ANTIDEPRESSANT?

"I'm at the end of my rope" . . . "Bad hair day" . . . "Got the blues" . . . "Down in the dumps" . . . are all expressions we use to describe a depressive episode. We all have had moments of depression in our lives, some have lived with it chronically. There are approximately 8 million women and 4 million men in the United States diagnosed with depression (Grant, 1994, p. 38).

At least two times more men than women are depressed for reasons for that have gathered much attention in the psychological community in recent years. Book stores have books that fill their shelves explaining the differences in women and men: *Men Are From Mars, Women Are From Venus, That's Not What I Meant, Men and Women.* One of the factors not often addressed in self help books is that of hormonal balance. Other reasons that have been explored are: cultural values that allow women to feel, while prohibiting men to do the same; women may just be more willing to admit that they are feeling depressed; men are more active physically and keep their biochemistry in better balance. Regardless, most people become dismayed when they realize that they have "fallen into a depression."

WHO IS DEPRESSED?

Research has indicated that among those women who are depressed, that single, divorced, and widowed women are less depressed than married women. However, conflicting evidence from other studies imply that married women are slightly less depressed than single women. Most studies agree that married women become as much as three time more depressed than single women if there are problems in their relationship (Grant, 1994, p.40).

Dr. Smith (1989, p. 93) found more men depressed during their mid 30's to age 40. He found that men, during this time period, began a reappraisal of their life's goals and progress. In that reappraisal period, he believes that men are confronted with an end of their "timeless idealizations" and their "boundless possibilities." Depression, for both men and women, is not just a day when you might be feeling low. It is diagnosed when it has persisted for a period of time.

SYMPTOMS OF DEPRESSION

Most professionals diagnose depression by listening to symptoms as reported by their patients/clients. Common symptoms, as listed in the *Diagnostics and Statistics Manual of Mental Disorders* (1987) are: loss of interest in previously pleasurable activities; feelings of worthlessness; feelings of excessive or inappropriate guilt; inability to concentrate or focus; lethargy, fatigue, or loss of energy; change in sleep habits, insomnia, extra need for sleep; change in eating habits resulting in significant weight loss or weight gain; feeling restless and unable to relax; feeling hopeless; difficulty making plans or decisions; unusual irritability; persistent physical symptoms, such as headaches, digestive disorders, or chronic pain; suicide ideation, thinking and/or planning to kill yourself or die. It is not that any of these symptoms are unusual in and of themselves. It is when five or more of these symptoms are present for at least two weeks that the diagnosis of depression is normally given.

Numbers of depression cases are climbing steadily among both men and women (also among some children and adolescents). Dr. Ellen McGrath, a clinical psychologist offered a well-rounded explanation for this: "Everyone is facing more economic uncertainty, and all of us are working harder and getting back less. Both men and women are faced with rapid changes in sex roles; men are now expected to be more emotional, while women have to deal with being in the workplace by choice or necessity. All these sources of stress can trigger depression" (Grant, 1994, p. 38).

WHAT CAUSES DEPRESSION?

There are many variables that can cause depression. Any situational stressor, such as the loss of a loved one, a divorce, or a change in job status, can result in a depression. There is also significant evidence that anger that is bottled up and turned inward (instead of appropriately dealt with) can result in depression. Biochemical imbalances can certainly cause depression, although there are those who believe that it is depression that causes the biochemical imbalances. Hypoglycemia and hypothyroidism can both cause depression. Alcoholism, drug dependency, or even addiction to prescription drugs can cause depression. In the many years I have seen patients in and out of hospital settings for depression, I have seen many who ended up depressed as a result of a dependency on a prescription drug they were taking as prescribed by their physician. Many times they would be in denial that such a thought was even a possibility. They became convinced when experiencing withdrawal symptoms when coming off the prescription. (Always to be done under the care of a physician).

Other causes of depression could include things such as: sugar dependency, glandular imbalance, or chemical and/or food allergies. In addition, negative emotions can disturb hormonal balances in the body, resulting in depression. This is only a partial list of possible causes of depression.

HOW TO HELP WHEN SOMEONE YOU KNOW IS DEPRESSED

Whatever the cause, depression is a "real" malady, not "all in the head" as has often been implied. I am approached on a regular basis by friends and loved ones of depressed patients wanting to know what they can do to help. I am amazed when I ask what they have done and find that most answers are similar: "I've told him to just snap out of it." Or "I keep telling her that she's just going to have to get over it." When someone says they are depressed, or express sadness or grief, the first thing they need is validation. "I know how hard this must be." Or "I hear that you are really struggling." The second thing you can do is to help them get into a mode of action. Whether that be to meet them for breakfast to help them get out of bed the next morning, or help them find a physician, or a good therapist, help them get into action.

TREATING DEPRESSION

There is a wide gap, even in the psychiatric/psychological fields, about what is the best method of treatment for depression. Some believe it to be a total biochemical problem, and believe that addressing the problem with drugs is the only option. Some believe it is a systemic problem which can only be dealt with by addressing the whole system. Others believe it is just a result of the way one thinks, and if he changes his thinking through a psychotherapeutic process, the depression will be alleviated. I prefer to think that there is validity in all of the above. If there are truly biochemical imbalances, those need to be addressed. (Although I don't believe the nearest prescription pad is always the best answer.) If there are systemic problems (problems in the marriage, in the family, in the workplace), those surely need to be addressed in a helpful setting. And certainly, the way we think and interpret events can have an impact on what we decide and how we feel about what we experience in life.

In his book, *Ageless Body and Timeless Mind*, Dr. Chopra states his beliefs that treatment with antidepressants does not cure the underlying sadness and that it was an ineffective method of treating depression. He believes "a more effective way to treat depression is through psychotherapy . . . Counseling a depressed patient, uncovering the inner hurt, and releasing it, sometimes accomplishes a lasting cure, which no drug can claim" (1993, p. 79). Psychotherapeutic processes (individual therapy, group therapy, marital therapy) and support groups no longer have the stigma attached that they once did. It seems that people are more willing to seek help when they need it.

Regardless of which avenue of help that is sought, it is important to seek treatment if the depression persists. Depression has appropriately been called the mood cancer because "it may spontaneously remit, but it will come back more severely [if nothing is done to diminish it]. Without intervention, it is guaranteed to get worse" (Grant, 1994, p. 40).

Before the prescription pad is reached for, I always hope that natural treatments are sought. The first scientific discovery that any mental illness might have a connection to nutrition and diet was when they discovered that pellagra (characterized by depression, diarrhea, and dementia) could be cured with niacin (Mindell, 1991, p. 238).

TREATING DEPRESSION NATURALLY

There are many natural foods, tips, and supplements that can be tried before prescription antidepressants. Vitamin B1 (thiamine) in above average does has been shown to help alleviate depression and anxiety attacks. Vitamin B6 (pyridoxine) aids in the production of dopamine and norepinephrine, our bodies' natural antidepressants. Vitamin C is able to help us combat stress. Vitamin B12 (cobalamin) relieves irritability, increases energy levels and improves our ability to concentrate. Choline has a soothing effect and folic acid has been shown to relieve depression. Zinc promotes mental alertness, which is often dullened while in a state of depression. Magnesium is an anti-stressor, and manganese reduces nervous irritability. Niacin is vital to the function of our nervous system. Calcium assists our bodies in relieving its tension.

Tyrosine, an amino acid, increases the rate at which our brain produces dopamine and norepinephrine, and phenylalanine helps our brain release them into our system once tyrosine has increased their production. Drinking bottled water is an important consideration for depressed people. Studies suggest that treated water can upset the balance of dopamine and norepinephrine.

Exercise, again, is of critical importance in depressed individuals. Dr. Kenneth Cooper, of the Cooper Aerobics Center in Dallas, Texas has developed and tested a method of exercising which has a major effect on all the body chemicals that play a role in depression. Dr. Cooper (1968) has noted that exercising for about thirty minutes four to five times weekly at your ideal heart rate can keep the body chemicals in balance and relieve depression.

In a study conducted using 67 men who were cardiovascular patients to determine the effect of an aerobic exercise program on their heart condition, an additional, unexpected benefit was noted. After a short time of aerobic conditioning, their depression began to lessen, they were more optimistic, had better insight into their personal problems, had improved self image and better self understanding (Hellerstein, et. al., 1967)

RESEARCH ABOUT DHEA AND DEPRESSION

In addition to these natural treatments, we once again turn to the use of DHEA, or a natural precursor of it. The literature is full of references to the impact of hormones on depression, much of it around females and menopause. It has been hypothesized that hormones influence behavior because their release (or lack of release) into the system causes emotional responses (Susman et. al, 1985). In support of that, adrenal activity has been shown to be decreased in subjects who were depressed (Janowsky et. al., 1987). Not only are the adrenals implicated in depression, but they are also implicated in anxiety, which can be an underlying symptom of depression. One study found that a decrease in the adrenal steroid revealed an increase in anxiety (Weiss, et.al., 1970).

The fact that depression is more prevalent in women supports the notion that the sex hormones play a role in some forms of depression. This is supported by the evidence that females with PMS (a condition where their hormones are out of balance) are at an increased risk for a subsequent major depressive episode (Glick, et.al., 1990). Natural progesterone, used to treat the PMS condition, is a natural mood stabilizer. This is further verified by noting that emotional depression decreases during pregnancy among significant numbers of women, a time when progesterone levels are naturally high (Glick, et al., 1990). Small pilot studies have also shown depressed patients improve when receiving natural hormonal supplements (Glick, et.al., 1990). In other studies, natural progesterone has been shown to relieve sad and negative feelings, and increase a sense of well-being (Cutler, 1990). One author, in reviewing the literature stated: "Studies show that hormone therapy can relieve depression that coincides with sex hormone deficiencies" (Cutler, 1990, p. 255).

There have been various studies which have investigated the impact of behavior on DHEA and DHEA-S levels, as well as the changes in the levels in the presence of certain stressors and events. One study noted that DHEA levels were high in females who had a high drive for activity and a high capacity for work (Hermida, et.al., 1985). Another study showed that an increase in DHEA resulted in improved task memory (Roberts, et.al., 1987). Another study demonstrated that exposure of male rats to the scent of female rats was related to changes in DHEA levels (Corpechot, et.al., 1985). These types of studies indicate that DHEA levels are affected in both cognition and motivation, both of which are factors in the behaviors of depressed people (Osran, et.al., 1993).

Research has also revealed that higher levels of DHEA were linked with people who were better able to express their anger (Inoff-Germain, et.al., 1988). This could be important when remembering that one of the possible causes of depression is when anger is unexpressed and turned inward. Perhaps that is simply a symptom of low DHEA levels.

Other factors and behaviors which could be related to depression have been noted in studies regarding DHEA levels. When exposed to chronic stress, it was noted that DHEA levels were significantly lower (Parker, et. al., 1985). Stress often leads to depression, and has been known to really put "wear and tear" on the adrenal system. When DHEA levels were lowered, the male aggressive response was significantly lowered as well (Haug et. al., 1989). Irritability is a symptom of depression, however, there is usually not enough to engage in an aggressive response when a person is in a depressive episode. Higher DHEA levels were correlated with higher risk taking behaviors in studying pilots in training (Klinteberg, et.al., 1992). It might be important to note that pilots who are depressed are not allowed to be admitted to training programs. DHEA levels are found to be low in boys who are hyperactive (Nottelmann, et.al., 1987). Many times, the symptoms for hyperactivity are misunderstood as "rowdiness," when it can actually be a state of chemical imbalance similar to that of depression. Some of the same prescription drugs used to treat hyperactivity are also used to treat depression and vice versa (i.e., prozac, dexedrine). When DHEA levels are down, some grandiose men tend to act out (Littman et.al., 1993). This concurs with the idea of many of the recovery authors who believe that grandiose acting out on the part of some men is their effort to conceal their pain and depression (Bradshaw, 1988). DHEA levels are also correlated with degrees of Type A behavior, characterized by being goal oriented, directed toward achievement with a sense of urgency, and easily annoyed if progress is impeded (Fava, et.al., 1987). Once again, the agitation described here is one typical in some forms of depression.

Few studies have been done using DHEA as a treatment for depression. However, many have directly correlated depression and DHEA levels. One particular study looked at DHEA levels from both sides of the coin. They began by assessing the depressed patients and noting that their DHEA levels were significantly low. They then used prescription antidepressants to relieve the depression. Subsequent testing revealed that the DHEA levels were also raised when the depression lifted (Tollefson, G.D., 1990). This study could add validity to the next four references regarding using a natural precursor complex to treat depression.

Parker, et.al. (1985) suggested that treatment through pregnenolone could provide the balance of corticoids and androgens that are necessary to cope effectively with stress and the ensuing depression. Recall that in the biochemistry chapter, we showed how the supplements made from saponins derived from Dioscorea villosa, the Mexican Yam, enter our system through the route of pregnenolone, making it the ideal supplement as described to be needed in the above study.

In the book, *Amazing Medicines The Drug Companies Don't Want You To Discover*, a study done by Dr. Bonnet is reported. He worked with a woman who had multiple diagnoses, one of them being manic depression. After low doses of DHEA for just one week, she reported feeling better. By the end of her treatment, she was able to begin and run a small business.

WHAT DOCTORS SAY ABOUT DHEA AND DEPRESSION

Another doctor recommends that the best treatment for depression is probably a natural progesterone and a low dose natural estrogen (Cutler, 1990, p. 261). Products that are derived from the Wild Yam and enter the system through the pregnenolone route are able to provide both!

Dr. Kamen (1993) finds that natural progesterone, when given to women for hormonal balance also serves as a mild antidepressant. Once again, the natural products, which can be obtained without a prescription, might serve as a natural antidepressant for both men and women.

Dr. John Lee of Sebastopol, California, in a telephone interview stated that he found natural progesterone products derived from the Mexican Wild Yam to be excellent treatment for depression. He delightfully explained that he did not begin using the natural progesterones with the expectation that they would bring about changes in depression levels. However, he began using it in treating some of his elderly osteoporotic patients. Soon after they would begin the

natural products, he would have their family members calling asking what he had done, or what miracle he had performed? When asking why the question, he would hear com-
ments like: "Well, she's balancing her checkbook, cleaning
house and taking care of things she hasn't done for year." Or
"He's happy and smiling all the time." It was then that he
began to note the natural antidepressant effect the natural products derived from the Wild Yam had on many of his patients
of all ages.

Depression is definitely NOT a welcomed guest when it
appears. A natural supplement would be a VERY welcomed
guest to many who suffer from depression, if it relieved their
symptoms.

COUPLE FINDS RELIEF FROM DEPRESSION!

Probably the most incredible story I have personally experienced is one of a patient of mine whom I will call Pat.
She came to me in a very depressed state for various reasons:
marital problems, financial difficulties, problems with her
children, problems with her aging parents. She came to me
at the referral of her psychiatrist who had tried her on several
rounds of various antidepressants without much change in
her mood. We began working through some of her issues,
and she experienced some relief. However, as I gathered her
history and found that she had had a hysterectomy several
years earlier, I conferred with her psychiatrist about a possible workup with an endocrinologist to determine hormonal
levels. She went for that evaluation and found that she had
some osteoporosis and was very low in some of her female
hormones.

I had informed her about some of the natural products
that were derived from the Mexican Wild Yam and she was
interested. After consulting with her endocrinologist and providing him with some information, he agreed to give her 30

days to try the supplements, then he would retest her. Long before her subsequent test, she was telling me she had not felt so good in ages. Not even since prior to her hysterectomy. "As a matter of fact, I don't think I've felt this good in my whole adult life." An interesting thing happened as a result in the change in her. Her husband, who was a skeptic of marital therapy agreed to come in for a session. We began resolving some of the marital difficulties and I noted that he, too, was suffering from depression. I recommended that he go for psychiatric evaluation, but that seemed a bit much for him. Several months later, as we were wrapping up the marital therapy, I noted his mood seemed much brighter and some of the depression symptoms I had noted earlier seemed to have subsided. When I asked him what he credited for that, he sheepishly smiled and said, "As soon as I found out those pills were not just for girls, I decided to give them a try myself."

10

DHEA AND THE LIVER:
THE HOUSE OF THE SOUL

Traditional Chinese medicine considered the liver to be the house of the soul. It was believed to be responsible for the flow of chi, energy, in the body. Linguists believe the word liver was derived from an Anglo-Saxon word "to live." Certainly "to live" . . . we must have well-tuned livers.

The liver is the largest gland in the body of all vertebrae animals. It comprises three to four percent of the total body weight of humans. The liver is a soft, solid organ, reddish brown in color, consisting of a right and left lobe, with the two smaller lobes on the lower back surface of the right lobe.

Blood flows to the liver directly from the heart, and also from the intestines. The blood oozes through some 50,000 tiny units called heptic lobules, about one millimeter wide. Here, chemical processes break down digested nutrients even further, assemble useful substances, filter old cells from blood, and store or release substances.

THE MANY FUNCTIONS OF THE LIVER

The liver is an essential organ which has more than 500 separate functions. Removal of the liver will result in death in one to five days despite attempts to replace the materials it produces. One of the major functions of this organ is the secretion of bile and its products. Bile salts and acids help emulsify fat, activate enzymes which digest fat, make fatty acids water soluble (required for absorption of fat-soluble vitamins), and exert antibacterial effects.

The liver serves as the center for the receipt and assimilation of foodstuffs, such as carbohydrates, proteins, fats, minerals and vitamins. It stores carbohydrates, regulates blood-sugar levels by the processes of glycogen synthesis and by breaking down glycogen to glucose. It is also the main site for the conversion of protein and fat to carbohydrates. Albumin and globulins (which are proteins not soluble in water) are synthesized in the liver, deamination, treansamination of amino acids is carried on, and urea is produced from ammonia. Fatty acids are metabolized, ketone bodies are formed, and cholesterol is produced in the liver.

The liver is largely responsible for detoxification. Drugs and substances which are potentially harmful to the body are converted into a water-soluble form and excreted into the bile, destroyed by liver cells, conjugated, or temporarily stored in the Kupffer or liver cells.

A variety of substances, including the Vitamin B complex and Vitamins A, D, and B12, copper, iron potassium, manganese, zinc, and cobalt are stored in the liver. Blood and water are temporarily stored here and released into circulation. The liver also produces clotting materials including prothrombin, thromboplastin, fibrinogen, and their precursors and activators. It also stores heparin and produces antithrombin and its analogous which prevent clogging.

THE LIVER PROVIDES THE BUILDING BLOCKS (PRECURSORS) FOR HORMONES

The liver is essential for healthy hormonal activity. The necessary precursors or building blocks needed for the production of hormones, and the enigmatic endocrine system are provided for by the liver. This liver activity plays a major role in hormone balance. The liver's hormonal precursors used by other hormone-producing glands are major factors in allowing the body to balance its hormone compliment. "A prehormone may be defined as an endocrine substance which has little or no biologic potency itself but is converted to more active compounds that mediate biological effects. DHEA is a sex steroid prehormone capable of being converted both to androgens and estrogens" (Leiter, et.al., 1987).

Several studies, especially those dealing with gynecological cancers, have identified a possible relationship between such cancers and unopposed estrogen, for example. Several of the sex-related hormones are produced directly by the liver. It is interesting to note that in the world of holistic, herbal medicine, many of the herbs used for the reproductive system are specifically indicated for the liver as well. Herbalists often include the liver as well as the reproductive system in treatment programs because such programs seem to create a synergistic effect.

DETOXIFICATION: THE MAJOR JOB OF THE LIVER

Perhaps the most important job of the liver is its role as the body's master detoxifier. It removes toxic substances from the bloodstream. Toxins either produced as a result of metabolism or absorbed from the environment are removed by a healthy liver. Even if they are eventually removed by a partially-functioning liver, if not removed in a timely manner, imbalances occur can cause both short and long-term health problems. Although any toxin can potentially damage the liver, it has considerable rejuvenating powers. The liver can function on a minimal level, even if 80% of its cells are damaged.

DHEA AND THE LIVER

"The findings of several researchers showing an inverse correlation between the urine levels of several hormones and the incidence of breast cancer in women have generated considerable interest in DHEA, since these hormones are primarily derived from DHEA" (Casazza, et.al., 1986). Since the liver is so central to the body's response to virtually all biochemically active substances, investigators have begun looking at the effect of DHEA on the liver itself. Some of the most specific, physiologically significant changes caused by DHEA have been discovered in the liver.

One study found several changes to liver composition with DHEA treatment (Frenkel, et.al, 1990). The study was designed to define some of the basic mechanisms that may explain the beneficial chemopreventative effects of DHEA. Treatments produced several profound changes in the liver. These changes included increased liver weight, color change, an increased number of peroxisomes, more mitochondria per cell, and increased levels of enoyl-CoA hydratase. These changes were found to be almost identical to those produced by compounds called "peroxisomal proliferators." Peroxisomal proliferators are widely believed to produce hypotriglyceridemia, a lowering of blood triglyceride levels. Reductions of between 18% and 27% have been observed in blood triglyceride levels (Stegmeir, et.al., 1982). Peroxisomal proliferations are widely believed to exert a cholesterol-lowering effect on the body. Reductions have been reported between 15% and 50% in rats, and 4% in humans.

Another study found significantly higher liver weights (as much as 65% higher) with DHEA treatments (Leighton, et.al., 1987). The researchers postulated that there was an increase flux of fatty acids through several liver pathways resulting in fatty acid synthesis. In layman's terms, Leighton proposes that this would constitute a substantial "energy wasting" system. Such energy wasting could explain the weight loss of laboratory animals receiving DHEA treatments.

Experiments were conducted to determine the structural changes in the liver that produced the results outlines in the liver studied mentioned (Bellei, et.al., 1992). The histological organization of liver of DHEA-treated rats was on the whole unchanged from that of the controls. However, the size of the hepatocytes was significantly larger in the rats fed DHEA. The DHEA treatment induced a significant 20% increase in mitochondrial proteins with no change of the glutamic dehydrogenase activity expressed per gram of liver. Fatty acyl-CoA oxidase, an enzyme also localized in peroxisomes, was 4-5 times greater upon short-term DHEA treatment. When rats were treated with the same dose of DHEA for 100 days, mitochondrial structure in the hepatocytes was altered. The mitochondria were characterized by a very dense matrix in which vacuoles were often observed. The ultrastructural transition of mitochondria is known to be associated with parallel functional transition from low rate to high rate respiration. The researchers stated that on the basis of the information available, it was not possible to determine whether the primary effect of DHEA is directly on peroxisome syntheses or on fatty acid mobilization that in turn might induce peroxisonal synthesis. The findings regarding the effects on the hepatocytes of rats subjected to long-term DHEA treatment are more difficult to interpret. The early effect on peroxisomes tends to decrease so that the number and the shape of peroxisomes tend to revert to those of control rats.

It is clear that the liver is directly affected by DHEA, perhaps more than any other part of the body. Because of the liver's central importance to our body's functioning, these changes, which appear to be much more positive than negative, are important indicators of DHEA's central importance to our health.

11

THE DEVASTATIONS OF CANCER, THE PROMISE OF DHEA TREATMENTS

Possibly the most dreaded three words in the English language are: "You have cancer." It is heard by hundreds of thousands of Americans each year. For some half million each, their dread becomes a reality. In the end, after a horrifying period of often degrading treatment, family members and friends must say goodbye to their loved one. Cancer, and its aftermath, touches us all.

A simple definition of cancer is that it is the abnormal growth of cells. The abnormal growth eventually interferes with normal bodily functions, and if not stopped, we die from the disease. Cancer begins with normal cells that change, although we are not quite sure why this happens. It is the cause that we ardently hope to find with all of our research. This change in normal cells, for whatever reason it happens, causes an increase in the rate of cell multiplication and a loss of cell differentiation.

There are two major theories about why cancer develops. Since cell growth and replication is controlled by DNA, one is a genetic theory of cancer that proposes that the cancer cell is a product of DNA damage. (DNA are our cells that carry our genetic makeup.) Since the likelihood of such damage increases as we age, the fact that cancer is more likely as we get older supports this theory. The second theory notices the link between cancer and toxic substances. These substances cause undamaged DNA to switch to this more primitive mode as a response. This theory is actually the more hopeful of the two. The correction of the cell's environment may lead to nontoxic treatment of cancer.

THE TRAGEDIES OF CANCER

Breast cancer is diagnosed in nearly 200,000 women in the U.S. each year. As many as 40% of these women will eventually die of the disease. Lung cancer, virtually the sole province of males before 1960, has now surpassed breast cancer as the biggest killer of women. "You've come a long way baby!" the cigarette slogan proclaimed a number of years ago. We certainly have, but the long way we have come is not a pretty picture. Colo-rectal cancer claims 150,000 victims each year, with prostate cancer not far behind in men. While gynecological cancers have become one of the few bright spots, with most curable if detected early, skin cancers have become far more prevalent as our worship of the sun continues.

Tens of billions of dollars and a huge industry, that employs over 800,000 full time, are engaged in our "war on cancer." Although at times it seems we are making progress, and we are on some narrowly defined fronts, the advances are slow and disheartening. The business is so large that the politics of money inevitably come to dominate the decision making process. The wars among the major players in the cancer field is usually kept behind the scenes, but hurts the efforts all the same. The National Institutes of Health, the National Cancer Society, and the National Cancer Institute fight for government and private dollars.

TOXIC TREATMENTS FOR CANCER PREVAILS

Although the fight for financial support for their studies to develop treatments continues, the same basic view of the disease and how to treat it remains in sync. To all of these groups, cancer is a localized disease represented by a tumor. Cutting it out, poisoning it, or irradiating it is the focus. Too often, treatments that are noninvasive and nontoxic, and thus nontraditional, are not only overlooked, but sometimes are ridiculed as well. The cancer industry does not want to hear about therapies that cannot be patented and thus kept proprietary . . . and of course the bottom line is . . . PROFITABLE! Dr. John Lee (1993) very candidly expresses his views regarding this matter: "It is interesting to note that only in the last five to six years has the U.S. cancer establishment recognized the importance of diet to cancer. It is now generally admitted that at least 35% of our cancer results from improper diet. Chances are the association is considerably higher than that. Yet, in U.S. cancer research funding, the proportion budgeted for nutritional research is only 5%" (p.79). Of course, there is no profit in treating cancer with appropriate foods.

This is not to suggest, however, that cancer researchers are not genuinely interested in and concerned about finding cures for cancer. It is simply to suggest that they are primarily interested in their cures being the one to be christened as "THE CURE."

DHEA AND CANCER PREVENTION

DHEA has been shown to inhibit cancer growth. Several theories have been postulated about how DHEA works. It appears to block the growth of carcinogens, and may slow the production of free radicals that have been shown to be involved in the formation of abnormal cells. Researchers have suggested that the metabolic changes attributed to DHEA may also be involved in its anti-cancer mechanism. It is speculated that the inhibition of the utilization of glucose, which is known to prolong the life of lab animals, may be one of these mechanisms.

BREAST CANCER

Breast cancer is the most written and talked about of all cancers, particularly in the popular press, such as ladies magazines, home magazines, and on television talk shows. If a first-degree relative (such as a mother, or a sister) has had breast cancer, the individual is twice as likely to develop the disease. This relationship is even greater if the relative developed the disease before reaching age 50. Of course, age is another risk factor in and of itself. Sixty-six percent of breast cancers are discovered in postmenopausal women. There are other risk factors as well, however, they are not as universally accepted. They include such things as: a high-fat diet, obesity, hormonal factors. Breast cancer is higher for women who have never given birth and among those who give birth to their first child after the age of 30. Menstrual history appears to be quite significant in evaluating risk factors. Early menopause, naturally occurring or the result of surgery, decreases the risk. The links between estrogen therapy, oral contraception, and breast cancer remains controversial. Breast cancer is one cancer where, other than avoiding dietary fats and controlling weight, lifestyle modifications do not significantly lessen the risk. By far the most important active measure is to focus on early detection. Adult women should train themselves to perform self-examinations, and they should have a baseline mammogram between the ages of 35 and 40. A mammogram every two years between the ages of 40 and 50, and then annually after age 50 is absolutely essential.

DHEA AND BREAST CANCER

DHEA has been shown to be an inhibitor in the growth of breast cancers. One study measured the hormone levels in 15 women who subsequently developed breast cancer, and then compared those levels to 29 matched controls from the same group of volunteers. The DHEA levels in the cancer group was 10% lower than in the controls. Among women who had had at least one child, DHEA levels were 17% lower among the cancer group (Helzlsouer, et.al., 1992). Two studies found that women with either advanced or primary operable breast cancer had low blood plasma levels of DHEA and DHEA-S (Wang, et.al., 1974; Zumoff, et.al., 1981). A study conducted on the island of Guernsey found that among 5,000 women aged 30 to 59 years old, those with either advanced or primary operable breast cancer had significantly lower levels of DHEA and DHEA-S (Bulbrook, et.al., 1971).

CANCER, SEX HORMONES, AND DHEA

Prostate cancer may be the most common cancer in males. The prostate is a male sex gland located beneath the bladder. It performs two major functions: first, as a valve insuring that urine or sperm flow in the proper direction, and secondly, as the maker of the white ejaculatory fluid in the male. It is dependent on the male hormone, testosterone, for its proper function.

Prostate cancer is primarily a disease of older men, with only 2% of patients under 50 years of age. After age 50, the rate of prostate cancer rises faster than any other cancer. Black males show a higher incidence of prostate cancer than do white males. Although common in the Americas and Europe, prostate cancer is rare in Asia. The fact that Americans of Japanese descent suffer much higher rates than Japanese indicates a strong dietary component of the disease.

A new screening test for prostate cancer, called the Prostate Specific Antigen (PSA) test, has been developed. This antigen is produced by a normal prostate gland. Blood levels of PSA generally rise as men get older and after massage or manipulation of the prostate. Blood levels also usually rise with prostate cancer. Although the PSA test misdiagnoses 20 to 35% of the time, it is still an excellent screening test for the more comprehensive transrectal ultrasound and needle biopsy tests. As usage of these multiple test techniques has increased, some interesting facts have become apparent. Miscroscopic cancer is detected in 41% of men between the ages of 40 and 49, and the percentage of men with this cancer rises with age, likely reaching 80% in men over 75. Whether these microscopic cancers are of real concern is debatable. In a European study, where such patients over 70 were divided into two groups, one receiving therapy and one simply being monitored, there was no difference in death rates (Lee, 1993).

GYNECOLOGIC CANCERS

Gynecologic cancers, cancer of the uterus, cervix and ovaries, are diagnosed 75,000 times each year in the United States. Among women who go through the proper preventative measures, regular exams, etc., uterine and cervical cancer are subject to early detection and have a relatively high cure rate. Ovarian cancer is often silent and deadly, particularly among women not paying attention to subtle changes in their bodies.

Of course, there is a hormonal connection to the cancers of the reproductive systems discussed above. Breast cancer is more likely in premenopausal women with normal or high estrogen levels and low progesterone levels (Cowan, et.al., 1981). This situation is most common after age 35. It is also common after menopause when women are given estrogen supplements without progesterone. Pregnancy, particularly early pregnancy, confers some protection. Men treated with estrogen (for prostatic cancer) have a higher incidence of breast cancer also. Prostate cancer, as eluded to earlier, has been associated with high levels of the predominant male hormone, testosterone.

Dr. John Lee, in his book, *Natural Progesterone* (1993), postulates that unopposed estrogens play a large role in such cancers. He strongly suggests using a different hormonal regimen in treating the loss of organs responsible for hormonal production other than the use of estrogen. He suggests using estriol and progesterone, two beneficial and safe hormones in such supplementation instead. Lee is also skeptical of the proposed relationship between testosterone and prostate cancer.

Given the various steps on the hormonal pathway when a natural source of DHEA is administered, it is clear that such a balancing effect can be achieved hormonally. Natural-source DHEA (not simply the synthetic drug, which should be avoided except under the close supervision of a physician very familiar with the product), comes through DHEA precursors. These precursors pass through several hormonal steps as they are naturally used by the body. If the material is available, the body will naturally select the various hormones it needs for its benefit.

DHEA'S EFFECT ON CANCER IN ANIMAL STUDIES

DHEA's effect on various cancers has received wide and varied study by researchers. A diet of DHEA has been shown to inhibit the development of thyroid tumors and liver lesions in rats (Moore, et.al., 1986). DHEA has also been shown to inhibit the appearance of invasive tumors of the colon, and of microscopic precursor lesions in mice (Nyce, et.al., 1984). Rats fed for several weeks a diet that contained DHEA had a reduction in the incidence of liver hemangiosarcoma (Weber, et.al., 1988).

The study of how DHEA works to provide this apparent anti-tumor effect has focused primarily on the evaluation of metabolic effects of the hormone. Most of the attention has been directed at a glucose utilization promoter called G6PD (glucose-6-phosphate dehydrogenase). Since the 1930s, researchers have known that this biochemical is present in significant quantities in many carcinomas. DHEA has been found to be an inhibitor of G6PD. The major role of reduced G6PD activity in the decrease in carcinogen metabolism has been demonstrated in several studies. In addition, some experimental evidence shows that inhibition of tumor promotion by DHEA may be correlated with inhibition of DNA synthesis (Feo, et.al., 1981, 1984,).

These results from researchers all over the world over a considerable period of time strongly support the existence of an anti-tumor effect of DHEA. The anti-tumor activity has been linked to several biochemical mechanisms, not the least of which is the inhibiting effect on G6PD. This research continues and the results could be life-changing for all those in the search for tools to fight this dreaded disease.

12

AGING, MEMORY AND ALZHEIMER'S DISEASE: HOW DHEA CAN HELP

Dr. John Lee (1994) of Sebastopol, California summarized it well in a paper in progress by saying: "Aging is as inevitable as death and taxes . . . " (p. 1). The truth is, with each day, we all age. However, it does not have to be a negative experience. As Dr. Lee goes on to say, " . . . but the prevention of premature aging is a goal to which we all should (and can) aspire" (p.1).

THE FOUNTAIN OF YOUTH

I remember a trip to St. Augustine, Florida in the late 1970's when I went with a group to the place discovered by Ponce de Leon which he hoped to be the Fountain of Youth. People by the bus load were going into that park to hear the lecture in a musty cave-like room, and get a small cup of the water coming from the spring. Everyone wanted to act like it was a silly, yet no one refused to accept, or drink, from the little white cup given them. The fountain of youth . . .

"Since ancient times, people have searched for the Fountain of Youth – a miracle fluid or substance that would roll back the years. How they longed to renew their youth, strength, vitality, to continue to be productive and to be free from degenerative diseases - heart attacks, stroke, arthritis (rheumatism back then), diabetes and cancer. They wanted to retain an accurate memory, sharp and quick thinking and positivism. And today we are no different" (Langer, 1994, p. 32). No different indeed!

Yet, it is amazing that we have information, as is seen in the pages of this book, that informs us that there is a substance, now available in natural form, which addresses almost every concern mentioned in the above paragraph. Dr. Whitaker (1992, p.1) must have realized this when in his newsletter, *Health and Healing*, he stated: "Ponce de Leon might still be here, if on his search for the fountain of youth, he had run across capsules of DHEA."

THE SEARCH FOR YOUTH AND LONGEVITY GOES ON AND ON . . .

Yet the search goes on. As the Baby Boomers reach middle age and face the aging process, longevity has become a hot topic in magazines, on talk shows, and in the medical community (Pizzorno, 1994, p. 30). Hopefully the talk will keep us more sensibly directed than efforts throughout the years have. The stories recorded in history regarding what physiologists, scientists, surgeons, and others have done to prolong life are astounding. One physiologist, Charles Edouard Brown-Sequard, tried to rejuvenate himself by injecting himself with the extract from a dogs testicles. Though claiming to be revitalized, he died several years later. Dr. Serge Voronoff, a European scientist, made millions of dollars performing testicular grafts from young monkeys. His claim to fame was supposed to be restoring youth, but became how he transferred syphilis from the monkeys to his patients. Dr. Paul Niehans, a Swiss surgeon, injected cells from the organs of the fetus of a sheep to rejuvenate the aging. His clinic may still be in operation, however, results are questionable (Airola, 1982, pp. 9-10).

All over the world, different cultures and groups have tapped into some phenomenal rejuvenating secrets. For example, Russia has found anti-aging properties in natural, raw unprocessed honey, Finland uses hyperthermia (hot saunas) to restore youth, Mexico holds the herb sarsaparilla as their miraculous rejuvenator. Each of these probably hold some value. One that holds value because of its results, is the secret of GotuKola used in China. This is a small plant found growing in the jungle of the Orient. It was highly proclaimed as a rejuvenator by Professor Li Chung Yun, who died at age 256.   He outlived twenty three wives and was still giving lectures at the University shortly before his death. He still had his natural hair and teeth at the time of his death, and many said that he appeared no older than a fifty year old man (Airola, 1982, pp. 111-112).

HOW LONG CAN WE LIVE?

Remaining healthy, full of life and vitality is of greater interest as our life span increases. At the end of the 1800's, the life expectancy was age 45 (Baulieu and Kelly, 1990, p. 144). In 1955, it had increased to 68.5 years and in 1993, it was 72 for males and 79 for females (*Amazing Medicines*, 1993, p. 275). Experts believe that our real biological lifespan capacity is 120 (Pizzorno, 1994, p.30). In Amazing Medicines the Drug Companies Don't Want You to Discover (1993), an article from the *Chicago Tribune* was reported to have contained an article by Dr. West where he predicted that new discoveries about manipulating genes that control aging could eventually extend life spans to 200, 400 or even 500. But just keeping it modest, if we can live to be 120, perhaps we need to rethink labeling someone who turns 30, 40, or even 50 "over the hill." It could be that it will not be until 60 that we are even "approaching the hill" if advancements continue and life spans increase.

ABOUT OUR WONDERFUL SENIOR CITIZENS

Our country tends to have a negative opinion of our aging, and of aging women more so than aging men. Our society seems to label our aged as "spent, sexless and senile." Yet a recent survey reveals that at least half of all Americans who are between the ages of 74 and 85, and also one third of the three million people who are over age 85 are HEALTHY AND ENERGETIC! Our attitudes toward our elderly might need some reexamination. In other cultures, the elderly are honored as wise, their advise is sought, and they are treated with great respect. In America, we tend to believe what science has reported: As we age, our brains shrink and by age 30, we begin a decline in neurons, and therefore, a decline which leads to memory loss, decreased reasoning abilities, and a reduction in our intellectual abilities (Chopra, 1990, p. 25).

However, research bears a different tale, a tale that renders those time honored scientific assumptions inaccurate. Studies indicate that healthy elderly individuals suffer from no significant memory loss if they are not lonely, depressed, or void of outside stimulation. In addition, research has indicated that their long term memory can improve. In a test where 70 year olds were compared with 20 year olds, the older performed better than the younger in long-term memory. Then after an opportunity to practice some short-term memory skills, the older group could almost match the young group in those skills (Chopra, 1990, p. 25).

CAUSES OF PREMATURE AGING

Age is not the enemy that we all fight, it is the degenerative diseases that accompany aging that become the real enemy (Rector-Page, 1992, p. 131). We can prevent those diseases by addressing the reasons/causes for disease and for premature aging: reasons and causes such as vitamin and nutritional deficiencies, poor diet, dehydration, alcoholism, cigarette smoking, use of illegal drugs (including marijuana), and exposure to environmental toxins (Rector-Page, 1992, p. 131; Lee, 1994, p. 15; Chopra, 1990, p. 27). Then ,there are the psychological and spiritual aspects which have everything to do with aging. However, it is difficult to make money promoting such changes in lifestyle, so fads about aging and longevity may always come and go (Airola, 1982, p 10).

NATURAL TREATMENTS FOR PREMATURE AGING

There are many natural remedies and preventions for aging. Some of the general ones include focusing on nutritional quality, instead of quantities of food eaten. As our metabolisms slow, fewer calories are needed, therefore, what we eat becomes of great importance. To accomplish this, it is recommended that smaller meals be eaten, avoiding fried foods, red meats, and highly processed foods. In addition, it is recommended that they keep their systems alkaline (by consuming lots of fresh veggies and whole grains), that they consume oceans foods several times weekly (for thyroid and metabolic balancing), that they eat cultured foods such as yogurt, sauerkraut, and tofu (to promote better nutrient assimilation), and drink plenty of bottled or mineral water daily. It is ideal for the elderly to weight between 10 and 15 pounds less than they weighed in their mid 20's (Rector-Page, 1992, p. 131).

To keep the immune system strong so that it can fight disease, these herbal supplements are recommended: bee pollen, Dong Quai, Siberian Ginseng, Ginkgo Biloba, Gotu kola, Dr. Chang's Long Life Tea, CoQ 10, Pycnogenol, Germanium, Vitamin E with Selenium, Chaparral and Fo Ti (Rector-Page, 1992, p. 131; Mindell, 1992, pp. 71-72, 96, 103). Ginkgo Biloba has been shown to slow the aging process, as has chaparral (Mindell, 1992, pp. 72, 103). In Louisville, Kentucky, a biochemist performed an experiment on mosquitoes and found that he could double their life span by supplementing them with Chaparral (Mindell, 1992, 71-72). Fo Ti, a Chinese herb, is considered to be a rejuvenating tonic. "The Chinese claim that Fo Ti can prevent hair from going gray as well as prevent other signs of premature aging" (Mindell, 1992, p. 96).

One of the most important aspects to consider in aging and longevity is exercise. Daily walks can assist the aging process in several ways. It can help a person maintain their ideal body weight and it can help provide the brain with the fresh oxygen supply it needs. Research indicates that those people who keep themselves in a moderate, regular exercise program have a longer life expectancy than the sedentary (Pizzorno, 1994, p. 32). In a recent article in a health magazine, Dr. Aesoph (1994, p. 37) states that "those who begin exercising later in life can slow or even reverse organ deterioration." According to her statement, it is NEVER TOO LATE to get started.

My mother is 65 years old and she began a walking program several years ago. She walks approximately10 miles daily, at a pace that others feel a need to jog to keep up with her. She is one of the most lively women of her age around, full of vitality! Exercise is a MUST for us all . . . but particularly, for us as we age.

USING MEDITATION TO STAY YOUNG

"The human body is designed for rejuvenation at any age, because youth is not a chronological age. It is a state of good heath and optimistic spirit" (Rector-Page, 1992, p. 131).

A good, optimistic spirit is more important than you might expect. "Research shows a pessimistic outlook on life depresses both personality and immune response" (Rector-Page, 1992, p. 131). It has been said that aging is a state of mind, and there is truth in that statement! One of the ways known to keep the mind positive, clear, and refreshed is daily meditation.

The psalmist David wrote in Psalms 119 ""'Oh, how I love your law! I meditate on it all day long. They make me wiser than my enemies, because they are my constant guide. Yes, wiser than my teachers...they make me even wiser than the aged." (Psalms 119:97-100, *New International Version and the Living Bible*). Since the beginning of time, meditation has been a prized activity of the wise.

In a research project, it was determined that meditators were younger biologically (as measured by blood pressure, acuteness of hearing, and near-point vision) than their chronological age. Those who have been meditating five years or less tested to be five years younger biologically than their chronological age. Those who had been meditating for more than five years tested to be twelve years younger biologically than their chronological age. (Chopra, 1990, p. 194).

Another study was conducted by Blue Cross/Blue Shield in Iowa with 2,000 meditators. Those who meditated regularly were hospitalized 87% less often than those who did not meditate. They also had significantly less problems with heart disease, respiratory ailments, digestive problems, and depression (Chopra, 1990, p. 194).

As mentioned in the chapter regarding menopause and hormonal replacement therapy, some people mistakenly believe that the older one gets, the less sexual activity the should or are able to participate in. However, Rector-Page (1992, p. 131) dispels that myth by advising "Enjoy a regular sex life. (Endocrine activity keeps you young.)"

That sometimes is difficult for the aging who "find themselves losing energy, retaining fluids, fighting fat, developing wrinkles and facial hair, prone to headaches and depression, and less interested in sex" (Lee, 1994, Paper in Progress, p. 13). The aging see doctors for medications that address symptoms only; they see cosmeticians to learn new make up tricks to "cover up" their age; they seek out surgeons for face lifts, tummy tucks, and liposuction; they seek out beauticians who can show them styles to hide their thinning hair, or get hair pieces and/or wigs; they read books about their loss of libido (because that certainly isn't kosher to talk about); they try to catch naps to conceal their fatigue, lack of energy, fading zest; they do almost anything to cope with the changes in their body, mind and spirit which are so spurned by our culture.

DHEA: YOU CAN STAY YOUNG!

Yet all the symptoms above can be addressed by a healthy lifestyle, exercise, good nutrition, some of the supplements listed, and by a natural supplement which is a precursor to DHEA!   Dr. Atkins clearly advocates this with his statement: "I strongly believe that using DHEA will improve your health and extend your life" (1994, p. 1).   Dr. Ward Dean makes a similarly strong statement: "DHEA levels naturally drop as people age, and there is good reason to think that taking a DHEA supplement may extend your life and make you more youthful while you're alive" (Dean, 1990, p. 95). That sounds pretty to close to the Fountain of Youth!

Countless articles and textbooks explain how DHEA levels peak at about age 20, and then begin a steady decline until there is little or none at time of death in the elderly. In an article published in the *New England Journal of Medicine*, a study revealed that DHEA is the predictor of life expectancy and age (Barrett-Conner et al., 1986). Another study which examined the role of DHEA in aging found that it was not only a marker of age, but it provided great opportunities for future studies if supplementing it could alter the natural progression of aging and its diseases (Regelson et. al., 1988).

More recent studies have made more bold statements about DHEA and the aging process. In a study using older animals, it was noted that changes in the dysregulation of immune systems in the elderly can be reversed when supplemented with DHEA (Weksler, 1993).

Studies regarding memory and old mice have been very revealing and hopeful. A group of researchers used mice to test the efficiency of DHEA in connection with memory. They put the mice in a maze that was shaped like a "T." They were trained to go from one part of the "T" to the other by a specific desired route by having an electrical shock applied until they got there after five seconds of trial and error. Once they learned the route, they were then injected with DHEA in differing amounts. All groups given DHEA showed significant enhancement of their memory retention. When given another drug which caused amnesia, those given DHEA still remembered the maze route. The implications of this research are that DHEA may not only enhance memory, but may alleviate amnesia (Roberts et.al., 1987). In another similar study using middle aged and old mice, "DHEA gave striking enhancement of memory retention" (Flood et.al., 1988, p. 180). Still another study revealed that memory was enhanced in both young and old mice using DHEA (Roberts, 1990, p. 13).

ALZHEIMER'S DISEASE

One of the major causes of institutionalization in nursing homes in the U.S. today is Alzheimer's disease. "This disease, characterized by progressive memory loss, confusion, and dementia, has risen in the last 20 years from relative obscurity to virtual epidemic proportions in the U.S. today" (Dr. Lee, Optimal Health Guidelines, 1993, p. 101). The disease was named in 1906 by a German physician, Alois Alzheimer, who studied the symptoms cluster and began using it as a diagnosis. In 1986, there were 2 to 2.5 million Americans afflicted with Alzheimers. By the turn of the century, that number is expected to double (Pelton, 1989, p. 298). The disease affects over 15% of the American population over age 65 (Nyholt, 1993, p. 21).

CAUSES OF ALZHEIMER'S DISEASE

The causes of Alzheimer's disease are varied and multiple. Rector-Page (1992) attempted to summarize the various causes. Some of those she listed studying various research included: poor or obstructed circulation, arteriosclerosis, anemia due to long or excessive drug use, decrease in hormone output, lack of exercise, lack of pure water, fluid accumulation in the brain, thyroid malfunction, aluminum toxicity (from aluminum cookware, deodorants, dandruff shampoos, anti-diarrhea medications, canned food, salt, buffered aspirin, fast foods), mercury toxicity (from silver amalgam dental fillings), genetic predisposition. About ten percent of the cases of Alzheimer's are found to be familial (Pelton, 1989, p. 293).

Autopsies performed following the death of Alzheimer's patients has shown an excess of aluminum, bromine, calcium silicon and sulfur in the brain. The same autopsies revealed deficiencies of boron, potassium, selenium, zinc, and Vitamin B12 (Nyholt, 1993, p. 22).

Dr. John Lee, in *Optimal Health Guidelines*, also points to food additives as a cause of Alzheimer's. He points out the danger of MSG which is a flavor enhancer used often in Oriental foods. He also mentions aspartame, which is in artificial sweeteners. He highly recommends avoiding both and warns that deceptive labeling may make it difficult to avoid.

NATURAL TREATMENT OF ALZHEIMER'S DISEASE

Rector-Page, (1992, p. 141) stated that "Natural therapies have been successful in slowing deterioration of brain function" and that "A highly nutritious diet is showing without question to be a deterrent of onset". She recommends following a hypoglycemia diet, eating organically grown food, consuming lots of the following: eggs, soy, foods, sea vegetables, whole grains, fresh vegetables, fiber, foods rich in Vitamin B (to block aluminum toxicity), and foods rich in tryptophan (poultry, low fat dairy, and avocados). She advises avoiding fats, salts, and meat.

Other supplements might be helpful in treating the symptoms of Alzheimer's. Mindell (1992, p. 103) reported that Ginkgo biloba "may be useful to relieve symptoms of Alzheimer's disease." Nyholt (1993) recommended the same, along with Butcher's Broom, Kelp, Vitamin B complex, with additional B6, B12, Vitamin C. Vitamin E, Boron, Potassium, Selenium, Vanadium, Zinc, and Coenzyme Q10.

DHEA: "HORMONE FROM HEAVEN" FOR ALZHEIMER'S PATIENTS

Once again, natural DHEA supplements offer hope. As mentioned in the chapter on hormone replacement therapy, estrogen is made through both routes of the pregnenolone chain which is the pathway through which the natural DHEA supplements enter the body chemistry. A recent report in Prevention Magazine, appropriately titled "Hormones from Heaven," reported a study that found women who took estrogen were 40% to 60% less likely to develop the Alzheimer's disease (1994, p.30). Perhaps DHEA could have a preventative effect in women (and possibly men) as far as Alzheimer's disease is concerned.

A study examining DHEA levels in Alzheimer's patients revealed that the DHEA levels were significantly lower in women with Alzheimer's than they were in men with Alzheimer's (Leblhuber et. al, 1993). Another study showed that DHEA levels were 48% lower in patients with Alzheimer's than other patients the same age without the disease (Merrill et.al., 1990) so there is definitely a correlation between the disease and the absence of DHEA in the body. Another recent study compared 102 Alzheimer's patients in partial or total care with mild to severe dementia with non hospitalized 80 year olds. It was noted that those with Alzheimer's had significantly lower DHEA levels (Nasman, 1991).

Perhaps the most hopeful are those studies where long-sought after hope for the treatment of Alzheimer's is directly addressed. One study noted that "administration of DHEA or DHEAS may be helpful in protecting the microvasculature against degenerative changes when low blood levels occur" (Roberts et.al., 1990, p. 60). Perhaps early detection of the disease can stop the degenerative process. Dr. Ward Dean states: "DHEA protects brain cells from Alzheimer's disease and other senility-associated degenerative conditions" (1991, p. 95).

Truly, the social, economic and emotional dimensions of Alzheimer's disease are staggering. And "the stresses in caring for a patient with this disease are so great that the caregivers are often driven to the breaking point" (Pelton, 1989, p. 297).

A HEART BREAKING STORY TO LEARN FROM

Recently, I heard a young lady ask an owner in one of the companies that manufactures a natural precursor complex if this natural supplement she had heard about was "for real." I expected her to be interested in the products because of their ability to balance her hormones or increase her energy level. But the story she told was different than the owner expected to hear. She told the story of a woman that everyone in her family lovingly called "Mamaw." Her "Mamaw" had been the light of her life, as well as the light of the whole family, and everyone who knew her. She had watched her grandmother deteriorate into dementia to the point where she could no longer care for herself. The whole family was traumatized over having to place her in the care of a nursing home. "Mamaw" didn't want to go. She wanted to stay in her wonderful little country home on a red dirt road in Arkansas, she wanted to continue working her garden which she had done for years, she wanted to continue to go to church and minister in any capacity needed from Sunday School teacher to song leader. But she tearfully told about Mamaw's decline. She then revealed her real interest was in preventing anyone else in the family from going down the same degenerative path that ripped the hearts and souls of those who had watched her "Mamaw."

She was assured that the research held hope for those who might be genetically predisposed to the disease. With great gratitude and thanks, she asked for brochures about the products, and declared that every member of her family would be presented with the opportunity to take them.

Maybe we could all learn from the heart rending story of another family and do what we can to prevent it in ours!

13

DHEA: HOPE FOR AIDS PATIENTS?

AIDS, Auto ImmunoDeficiency Syndrome, has been called the most "complex disease organism ever discovered" (Chopra, 1989, p. 254). AIDS is not a single disease, but a constellation of symptoms believed to be caused by infections and/or cancers because of a disruption of the normal functioning of the immune system when taken over by a viral infection. When the immune system breaks down with the viral infection, the body becomes progressively unable to defend itself (Rector-Pate, 1992, p. 132).

THE CAUSE OF AIDS

AIDS is actually caused by HIV (Human ImmunoDeficiency Virus), a virus which infects the T4 blood cells and the macrophages, causing a reduction in the effectiveness of the body's immune system to fight disease and infection. ARC (AIDS Related Complex) is a term rarely used anymore, but was originally coined to refer to those AIDS patients who had less severe, less fatal symptoms. If untreated, it is believed that HIV patients will develop full blown AIDS within eight to eleven years. Further, it is also believed that with no treatment, 78 to 100 % of those with AIDS will die in

15 years (Douglas and Pinsky, 1992, p. 3).

VAST NUMBERS OF CASES REPORTED

"Unfortunately, in our generation we have witnessed the uncovering of one of the most chilling examples of a new disease in recent world history, AIDS" (Berger, 1988, p. 230). In the late 1970's, there were no reports of AIDS cases in humans. In 1981, when the Federal Centers for Disease Control (CDC) began monitoring for AIDS cases, there were few cases to be found in the U.S. Now, AIDS cases have been reported in all of the 50 states. In May of 1991, there were 1.5 million cases reported world-wide. In June of 1991, there were 179,136 diagnosed cases of AIDS reported in the U.S. (Douglas and Pinsky, 1992, p. 1). By the end of 1992, it was estimated that 365,000 would be diagnosed with AIDS (Douglas and Pinsky, 1992, p. 20).

ASTOUNDING NUMBERS OF DEATHS

The death rates predicted by this disease are astounding. Dr. Schepper (1993, p. 2) reported that by the year 2000, 1.5 million deaths in the United States were projected to be caused by AIDS. He also reported that by the same year, one-third of Africa's population was projected to be wiped out as a result of the disease. However, not just Africa and the United States are plagued with the disease. AIDS is becoming the number one health problem in Asia as well.

There are varied statistics regarding who dies in what time period once they have contracted AIDS. Chopra (1989, p. 252) in *Quantum Healing* stated that 80% of the patients diagnosed with AIDS die within in two years of their diagnosis. The disease is currently the leading cause of death among young men aged 25 to 44. Douglas and Pinsky (1992, p. 16), in *The Essential AIDS Fact Book* stated that more Americans would die in 1993 from AIDS than vets who died in action from the entire Viet Nam era.

AIDS EFFECTS BOTH MEN AND WOMEN

This disease is primarily a disease of the male gender, but females are not excluded. About 10% of the total AIDS cases reported are females, with 79% of those females being in the age range between 13 and 44. As of June 1991, 17,730 of the reported cases were women (Harding and Pinsky, 1992, p. 16). Among women, the incidence of AIDS was 12 times greater in black women and Hispanic women than in white women. In cases involving children, there was a 15 times higher probability of it being diagnosed in black children than in white children (Harding and Pinsky, 1992, p. 18).

Of those males that contract AIDS, approximately 54% are white, 29% are black, and 16% are Hispanic. Because blacks comprise 12% of the U.S. population and Hispanics comprise 6%, both groups are proportionately overrepresented as AIDS victims. In addition Caucasians who contract the disease have a life expectancy two to three times longer than for blacks (Harding and Pinsky, 1992, p. 18). The reasons for this may not be so much physical as socioeconomic. Treatment for AIDS patients is exorbitantly expensive, and those without appropriate health insurance may not get the quality of care, or may not be able to afford the quality of care that others get.

SYMPTOMS OF THE DISEASE

As stated earlier, it can be a matter of years between the time that the virus is contracted and the symptoms emerge. Some of the common symptoms are: fatigue, loos of appetite and/or weight, inability to heal minor ailments, night sweats, enlarged liver and/or spleen, skin disorders, recurring respiratory infections, and chronic diarrhea (Rector-Page, 1992, p.134).

Many of these symptoms in and of themselves are common. That is the reason for calling this virus a "syndrome." It is when they are experienced in clusters that there is concern. Douglas and Pinsky (1992, p. 57-58) state that the presence of the following symptoms are a good reason to consult with a physician:

- Severe dry cough or progressively worsening shortness of breath,
- Blurring of vision, "floaters," or loss of visual field,
- Colds or sore throats that persist for several weeks,
- Blood or mucus in the stool
- Liquid stool for five or more days, or loose stools for more than three weeks, or any loose stools accompanied by fever or weight loss,
- Headache for three days or more,
- Confusion or loss of memory,
- Localized unexplained muscular weakness,
- Fever, severe unexplained fatigue, or malaise,
- Drenching night sweats,
- Easy bruising or unexplained bleeding,
- Purplish or discolored areas on the skin,
- Unexplained loss of 10% or more of body weight,
- White creamy patches in the mouth
- Unexplained persistent swollen glands

People who contract the virus, may not actually develop AIDS, but that may dependent upon early diagnosis and preventative treatment.

HOW HIV INFECTS THE SYSTEM

The reason that symptoms of the virus often does not appear until months or even years after it is contracted is not fully understood. Perhaps the most simple explanation is that HIV blends itself into our DNA's chemical strands, masking itself as part of the host's genetic material. It then lies dormant until the DNA is triggered to produce antibodies to fight some infection or disease. The retrovirus then wakes up and begins to duplicate itself by the millions because it has joined itself to the DNA chemical strands that produce antibodies to fight off infection. (Chopra, 1989, pp. 253-254).

Once the virus has become AIDS, the most common cause of death in AIDS patients is opportunistic infections and cancers. Therefore, the reason for early diagnosis and preventative treatment is to stay strong, which reduces chances of succumbing to full-blown AIDS and/or other infections (Rector-_age, 1992, p. 133). Also, buying time is very important as research in this area progresses. It allows time for the research for a virus-inhibiting compound to progress.

NATURAL TREATMENTS FOR HIV AND AIDS

There are some natural treatments to which more and more HIV and AIDS patients are turning. In the field of herbal and homeopathic medicine, more hope is emerging for these victims. Rector-Page (1992, p. 133) stated: "Indeed there are enough success stories just in the last eighteen months from the people themselves, and the holistic practitioners working with them, to indicate that holistic therapies are showing more promise than ever. AIDS, ARC, and other immune deficiency diseases are no longer seen to be inevitably fatal as they once were. Holistic programs are frequently causing symptoms to abate and gradually disappear. The advance of the virus itself has been slowed in many instances, and improved longevity and quality of life are observed even in full-blown AIDS cases."

Although I am not in any way suggesting that HIV or AIDS patients should abandon their medical care, perhaps considering some of the natural methods of treatment would be worthwhile. Rector-Page (1992, p. 133) compiled the most common natural treatments recommended in the most recent edition (9th) of her book, *Healthy Healing, An Alternative Healing Reference*. The following is a summary of some of those recommendations as well as their purpose.

Megadoses of ascorbate Vitamin C crystals are recommended to flush and detoxify the tissues. Ten to twenty teaspoons daily for two to three weeks are recommended for the initial flush, followed by ten grams weekly. Vitamin E at 1000 i.u.'s daily is recommended for an anti-infective formula. This should be used with selenium and beta carotene at 100,000 i.u.'s daily.

Raw thymus extract three times daily has been shown to strengthen immunity. Echinacea extract at 1/2 a dropperful three times a day has been shown to stimulate production of interferon, interleukin, and lymphocytes. Because of this, Gladstar (1993, p. 29) stated that "Current research indicates that echinacea hold promise as an AIDS treatment." Shitake mushrooms are believed to achieve the same results. Other teas, seeped for thirty minutes which are supposed to have similar results on the stimulation of production of inferon, interleukin, and lymphocytes are as follows: prince ginseng roots, dry shiitake mushrooms, echinachea angustifolia root, schizandra berries, astragalus, ma huang, pau de arco bark, and St. John's wort.

Fresh vegetable juices made from organic veggies processed in a home juicer three times daily are recommended. Carrot, beet, and cucumber juice is strongly recommended in combination with garlic extract and flax oil for liver detoxification. Then chewing one to three DGL tablets is suggested to neutralize acids this might release in the system.

Drinking two to three glasses of aged aloe vera juice has been found to block the virus spread from cell to cell. Potent anti-oxidants, such as CoQ 10 (30 mg), Germanium (100-150mg), Pycnogenol (50MG. four times daily), Glutathione (50 mg. two times daily), or Octacosonal (100 mg. daily) have been noted for overcoming some of the side effects and some of the nerve damage cause by AZT. It also strengthens the white blood cells, and T-cell activity. This combined with Quercitin Plus with bromelain (500 mg. three times daily) has been indicated for improvement of the respiratory system.

Sun Chlorella at 15-20 tablets daily or two packets of granules daily have shown to build the immune system. Shark liver oil or shark cartilage (one 740 mg. caplet for every 12 pounds of body weight daily) taken for three weeks before meals, then reducing it to four to six caplets daily, has been shown to increase leukocytes and white blood cell activity, which fights infection.

AL721, an extract of egg yolk, has been used to treat AIDS patients successfully in Israel. According to Dr. Ward Dean, the preliminary research using AL721 conducted by the Israelis suggests that "it might eliminate some of the symptoms of AIDS" (1990, p. 93-43).

It has been suggested that taking weekly colonics will remove infected feces from the intestinal tract, keeping the infection from spreading further. Other natural treatments recommended included: macrobiotic diet with more raw foods, positive mind set through support groups, therapy, or biblio/audiotherapy, and plenty of rest and relaxation.

FACTS ABOUT AIDS

Much of our society remains uneducated about this disease, and therefore, prejudices and fears exist. AIDS and HIV are not airborne diseases, and therefore, cannot be caught in casual contact with those who have the virus. It is NOT spread by saliva sprays with sneezes, or coughs; it is not spread by drinking out of a water fountain after someone with the virus, nor from drinking out of their glass; it is not spread in tears nor in urine (for those afraid to use the restroom in public places); it is <u>NOT</u> spread by any casual contact.

The virus is primarily transmitted in three ways: 1) through any contact with sexual discharges or blood with mucous membranes, 2) through the blood (transfusions, sharing needles in drug use, etc.), or 3) from the mother to the fetus. According to current statistics, 63% of the transmission is through sexual contact, 28% is through needle-sharing, 3% is from blood transfusion, and 4% is unknown. Of the 63% reported to be from sexual transmission, 58% is from sexual contact between men, and only 5 to 9% is transmitted in sex between men and women.

PREVENTION OF AIDS

As some cases that have been publicized between physicians or dentists and patients indicate, we cannot be 100% safe from contracting the virus. However, these common safeguards are recommended: abstain from anal intercourse, practice safe sex, do not do intravenous drugs, and have all blood transfusions thoroughly checked when they are absolutely necessary. Of course, the safest sexual safeguard recommended is to abstain from sex outside a commited, monogamous marriage, and then be tested first if there has been other sexual contact.

AIDS PATIENTS TAKE CHARGE

When patients do get diagnosed with HIV or AIDS, probably no one knows the terror that grips their lives. Anyone who has had any significant contact with the gay male community is familiar with the terror and agonizing sorrow the disease brings. Perhaps it is this terror and agony that make so many AIDS patients adamant about seeking and getting the cutting edge treatments, whether they are known to be effective, or being researched to determine their effect. This is clearly demonstrated with the activist position that many

AIDS patients and their loved ones have taken with the FDA. In July of 1988, the FDA ruled that up to three months supply of drugs not approved in the United States could be shipped in for personal use. In Dr. Ward Dean's book, *Smart Drugs and Nutrients* (1990, p. 26), he reprinted an article as it appeared in the New York Times following the policy change of the FDA Pilot Guidelines Chapter 971, and it stated: "The new policy was the direct result of pressure from desperate AIDS patients, who have only one approved treatment available in the country, AZT, or azidothymidine, which is too toxic for many patients to take for long periods . . . "

As a result of their demands, non-profit organizations, such as the PWA Health Group, have been established to supply drugs for people with AIDS who have a hard time finding experimental treatments. There are many of these buyer's clubs set up for differing diseases in different parts of the country. Perhaps this is one of the most significant reasons for the development of a natural precursor product that could be helpful to these patients.

RESEARCH ABOUT DHEA WITH AIDS PATIENTS

Dr. Ward Dean stated that "DHEA is now being used by many people with AIDS because of its immune-enhancing and antiviral effects" (1990, p. 97). The research about the use of DHEA is somewhat sparse at this time, however, there is a positive tone to what is noted.

The AIDS Treatment News, in a 1988 edition, featured an article called: "DHEA: Mystery AIDS Treatment" (James, 1989, p. 236). It was called the mystery treatment because of the difficulty they had obtaining information regarding a study being conducted in Paris treating AIDS patients with DHEA. They found out about the study through several of the patients involved in the study. Apparently there were 10 people in the study, five of whom were American. The problem with obtaining results of the study seemed to be that the microbiologist who conducted the study in cooperation with a pharmaceutical company had experienced some disagreements. The subjects themselves believed that the microbiologist desired to publish the results quickly, but that the pharmaceutical company was anxious to create a variation of the drug which was patentable before releasing the research. When both parties were contacted regarding the study, one was legally forbidden to participate in the interview, and the other party denied the research had been conducted.

However, the *AIDS Treatment News Team* was able to locate six of the ten participants and consult with a number of other physicians regarding the results to present the information as best they could. Of the participants in the study they were able to interview, they obtained the following results:

One had his T cell count improve from 248 to 641, and his KS lesions seemed to be lightening. Another had slight improvement in T cell count, but other blood values which had been low had all moved into the normal range. In addition, his fungal infections and leukoplakia (precancerous change in mucous membrane, usually in mouth, causing thickened white patches) had all cleared up. Another had T cells count go from 186 to 560. His fungal problems also cleared up without the use of other medications other than the DHEA.

Another who was overweight at the start of the study lost weight and reported far more energy. The fifth male had started doing quite well, but withdrew from the study. The sixth wasn't doing well, but improved after a platelet transfusion.All six were given oral doses, 200 to 300 mg. daily, working up to 500 mg. daily, at 100 mg. five times daily before meals.

In speculating about the results, several scientists offered these explanations: DHEA has shown to have immune-suppressing effects on rats in clinical studies; DHEA may stimulate the bone marrow to increase production of red blood cells, platelets, monocytes, macrophages, and lymphocytes; DHEA may work by helping to bring all blood elements normally lower in AIDS patients back up to normal range (James, 1989, pp. 239-240). The conclusion of independent scientists reviewing this information was that DHEA may have a direct antiviral effect.

Persons with AIDS do have abnormally low levels of DHEA. In one study, designed to investigate the DHEA levels in connection with persons with HIV infection, it was found that: "The length of survival after the onset of initial AIDS symptoms is consistent with the normal plasma distribution of this steroid, in that the survival of older adults and young children in less than that of young adults" (Merril et. al, 1990, p.102). Another study observed twenty-three HIV patients taking DHEA for at least 16 weeks at very high doses. It was noted that DHEA inhibits HIV, and that the high doses were were tolerated by the patients (Dyner et.al., 1993).

NEW HOPE FOR AIDS PATIENTS

In 1991, the results of the San Francisco Men's Health Study concurred with the issues of DHEA levels and declining health in AIDS patients. This study involved 1034 single men between the ages of 24 and 55 years of age. The subjects were examined and tested at least every six months throughout the study. It was noted that there was a faster progression for HIV to AIDS in patients who have subnormal DHEA levels. They also reported that these results were " . . . consistent with in vitro and animal data that suggest a protective role for DHEA in viral infection" (Jacobson et. al., 1991, p. 867). Another study also indicated that DHEA could be effectively used to protect the system against lethal infections whether they were viral or bacterial (Loria, et. al., 1990, p. 125).

In an in vitro study (using human tissue in a lab setting), some other significant findings regarding HIV and AIDS were found. DHEA was shown to be an inhibitor of HIV replication in human lymphocytes (part of the white blood cell system which increase to fight infection). However, higher concentrations of DHEA were needed than the body normally produces. DHEA also inhibited HIV replication in human macrophages (cells that surround and destroy debris in the cells of the body) (Schinazi, et.al., 1990, p. 170).

At the Sixth International Conference on AIDS in 1990, a research study was revealed that involved thirteen patients that showed some immune function improvement with high doses of DHEA. There was also slight increase in T4 cell count in five of the patients (Smith, 1991). In addition, another study has shown that DHEA moderately inhibits the Epstein-Barr virus (Smith, 1992).

One patient, whom I will call Fred, was previously in the medical profession himself. He knew of the research being done, and as a result of early hope presented through the Paris study, began obtaining the drug. He has been able to maintain his T4 cell count steady for several years, which he attributes to the intake of DHEA. He is currently taking the natural product derived from the Mexican Yam, while having his blood levels checked regularly for DHEA and DHEA-S. The first month's reports showed his levels maintained with the natural precursor product.

Although the exact benefits of DHEA are still being thoroughly researched, several AIDS patients who had been obtaining the drug through what they call the "underground market" are reportedly now taking the natural precursor complexes and are pleased with the results.

14

THE MOST FREQUENTLY ASKED QUESTIONS ABOUT DHEA

QUESTION: If I take the natural products that are derivatives of the Mexican Yam, that can be converted to DHEA in my body, will it affect my thyroid medication?

ANSWER: The precurcor function of the dioscorea found in the Mexican Yam is important to this question. Hormone synthesis is a dynamic fluctuating system, responding to changing body conditions and needs. DHEA's level of activity is in response to the body's needs. It is controlled by the balance between its production from cholesterol and its metabolism and excretion by the liver. If thyroid activity is impaired, it is reasonable to assume that this natural source of DHEA may increase thyroid activity. You may need to lower your thyroid supplements. You should monitor your thyroid supplement needs with your health care provider.

QUESTION: How will I know if the recommended amount of DHEA is the right amount for me?

ANSWER: Again, using a natural precursor that the body can use for its needs is the important point. In general, your body tends to utilize the extra percursor to make DHEA if it needs it, and ignores the precursors if it doesn't.

QUESTION: What effect does alcohol have on DHEA levels?

ANSWER: Studies have shown that large differences in the levels of gonadal hormones occurs when alcohol is present. It is reasonable to assume that this mechanism is present with respect to these hormone's precursor, DHEA. It is likely that those who use alcohol more heavily will have lower levels of DHEA.

QUESTION: Is it true that DHEA can help in recovery from brain injuries?

ANSWER: Research on test animals has shown that pre-treatment with progesterone gives an extra recupretive boost to brain tissues. As a precursor to progesterone, DHEA is certain to show a like effect. Further strength is given to this position by the evidence of DHEA's positive effect on other neurologic disorders such as Alzheimer's disease.

QUESTION: I was hoping to lose some weight taking this product. Does everyone who takes it lose weight?

ANSWER: Unfortunately, not everyone does lose weight when taking the products derived from Dioscorea villosa, even though it has been shown to convert to

DHEA in the body, and research points toward weight loss with DHEA. Regelson et. al. (1988) reported in one of their studies that cancer patients who were supplemented with DHEA for two and a half years did not have substantial weight loss. However, as mentioned earlier, DHEA is called the "mother steroid." This is because it has no biological impact in and of itself, but it seems to know where it is needed in the body, and goes to that need. The cancer patient mentioned in the study above had significant results with their disease when on DHEA. Don't you think that that had more importance to their condition than weight loss? I certainly think they probably did. However, if you will stay with it, you may experience weight loss after other imbalances or abnormalities in your system are taken care of.

QUESTION: If I am not losing weight yet, do you have other suggestions about my weight?

ANSWER: This is a difficult question to answer, because we live in a "fast fix it" world where we want immediate results. First of all, don't try a fad diet, and don't starve yourself to death. One thing that we know is that you need to be eating foods that are right for your body and its system. Many programs encourage everyone to follow their menu, but the truth is, you need to be eating food in the right proportions for your body. The only way I know to accomplish that is to do metabolic balancing questionnaires. In the meantime, you can follow a moderate exercise program, eat healthily, and avoid fats and processed foods. Truly, when your body is in balance, and you are eating properly, there is no reasons these supplements should not assist your weight loss.

QUESTION: I am about forty years old and have lost weight and kept it off for a number of years. I began taking Emprise Plus, one of the Dioscorea products, and I actually gained weight for the first month. What on earth happened?

ANSWER: I spoke extensively with a colleague of mine who specializes in internal medicine and endocrinology. He advised me that if a female who takes these products is deficient in hormones, it begins to supply the body with long awaited and needed estrogens or progesterones. The body, much like when you begin to increase you water intake, seems to hold on to the hormones through fluids. However, just as when you continue to drink lots of water, your body will begin to release the fluid when it realizes it will continue to get it, your body will stop "holding" hormones which can cause a "false" weight gain that might feel like bloating.

QUESTION: I have heard that even if I have gone through menopause, I can start having periods again on these products. Is that true?

ANSWER: Increased levels of progesterone can cause some breakthrough bleeding, as the excess stored estrogen is released. But this should cease in a matter of a few months. If it doesn't, you will want to check with your physician. In addition, we have found that women who have experienced a premature menopause due to stress, medication or other unnatural causes have begun to menstruate again once their endocrine system becomes normalized. We are seeing this as a temporary state so far. However, the only thing to be disappointed about is the inconvenience. Just when you thought you were finished, here it all is again. Your body obviously was prematurely induced into menopause if this is the case and it could be normalizing itself. If it continues, you need to consult with your physician.

QUESTION: I understand that the supplements made from the Dioscorea extract can go through a pathway that can make estrogen. My doctor says that if I continue to have hotflashes, I will need some supplemental estrogen. Are there any other natural sources of estrogen?

ANSWER: As always, follow your doctor's recommendations. However, some writers, such as Airola (1982) have suggested getting natural estrogen from herbal supplements, such as : false unicorn roots, black cohosh, and elder flowers.

QUESTION: I have noted that females seem to have an "adjustment period" when they begin taking supplements made from the Wild Mexican Yam. Can you tell me why some of us women are experiencing that?

ANSWER: It seems that some women have a "detox" period of time, lasting anywhere from a few days to six weeks once they begin the products. There is nothing in the products that are natural that should cause adverse side effects, but remember that anytime your body gets what it needs, it has a tendency to go through a period of releasing toxins. Should adverse symptoms continue, check with your physician.

QUESTION: I have heard that you should not take these products if you have a history of prostate cancer in your family. Is that true? Why?

ANSWER: Studies have shown a link between high levels of the male hormone testosterone and prostate cancer. Although this link is disputed by some, it is generally accepted as true. Since natural DHEA precursors would normally act to increase testosterone levels, it would not be advisable to take precursor supplements if you have an inherited tendency to prostate cancer.

QUESTION: I have heard that these natural supplements which contain progesterone can cause males to have decreased sexual desire and functioning. Is that true?

ANSWER: When natural progesterone is taken by men under age 45, their libido can decrease. However, when taken by men over 55, the libido has been shown to increase. The one thing to remember about products that are taken through the pregnenolone route, it can convert to progesterone, but it can also pass through the DHEA route and convert to testosterone. As the "mother hormone", it should know which your body needs, and therefore, should not affect libido. If you do experience a drastic change in libido, or a prolonged slight change, consult with your physician.

QUESTION: Are there any differences in the DHEA levels of athletes and of others of the same age?

ANSWER: Studies have shown that the blood levels

of DHEA-S was significantly higher in athletes (Cacciari, et.al., 1990).

QUESTION: As an athlete, I can be disqualified from participating in sports if they find any steroids in my blood when tested. Can I take the Dioscorea product that one company calls "Sport" and be disqualified when tested?

ANSWER: No. Because this product does contain a natural source of the hormone precursors, the only "steroids" that testing would find would be naturally occuring ones, and at levels the body would produce. This is not the type of steroid abuse being tested for.

QUESTION: What is a thermogenic? And is DHEA a thermogenic?

ANSWER: "Thermogenesis" refers to the production of heat by the cells of the body. Increased thermogenesis produces more heat in the cells, which burns energy, which leaves less energy for the body to store as fat. Studies (Bobyleva 1993) have shown that DHEA enhances thermogenesis. It is speculated that several known biochemical mechanisms, including increased activities of cytosolic enzymes, contribute to this effect.

QUESTION: Do these naturally-occuring precursor complexes made from Dioscorea (the Mexican Yam) really raise blood levels?

ANSWER: A physician friend of mine, Ann (see more of her story in the chapter about diabetes) agreed to have her blood levels checked at an independent lab to determine whether or not the natural precursor products were actually raising blood levels. She had her DHEA levels checked in the middle of February before she began taking the product. But the middle of March, her DHEA levels had increased 46%, and by the middle of April, they had increased 91%. Several others have brought lab test results for me to review which also indicate that the products can raise DHEA levels in the body.

QUESTION: Does that thigh cream stuff really work?

ANSWER: A friend of mine, whom I lovingly claim as "my little sister," has used the thigh cream for several months now. She had been struggling for years with that "dimpling" effect that we all get on our thighs. Even when she got down to 105 pounds to compete for Mrs. American Queen (which she won in 1992-1993), she still struggled with the dimpling. However, with daily use, combined with the oral intake of the DHEA precursor, she reports delightfully that those old dimples are beginning to smoothe out. She is pleased that the thigh cream with the hormonal precursor, in combination with the oral precursors, seem to provide more than the mere cosmetic effect that the aminophyline products provide.

APPENDIX A

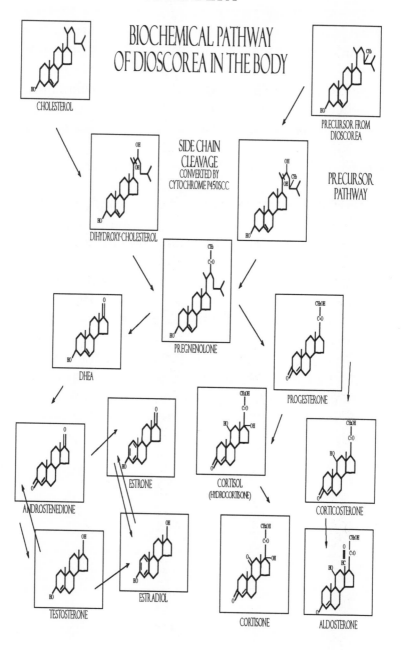

BIOCHEMICAL PATHWAY OF DIOSCOREA IN THE BODY

CHOLESTEROL

PRECURSOR FROM DIOSCOREA

SIDE CHAIN CLEAVAGE
CONVERTED BY
CYTOCHROME P450SCC

PRECURSOR PATHWAY

DIHYDROXY-CHOLESTEROL

DHEA

PREGNENOLONE

PROGESTERONE

ANDROSTENEDIONE

ESTRONE

CORTISOL (HYDROCORTISONE)

CORTICOSTERONE

TESTOSTERONE

ESTRADIOL

CORTISONE

ALDOSTERONE

APPENDIX B
THE BIOCHEMISTRY

Although about 50 steroids have been isolated from the adrenal, few have significant hormonal activity and few are secreted in any significant amount (Granner, 1988). The adrenal produces these hormones from three different zones: the zona glomerulosa, the zona fasciculata, and the zona reticularis. Bothe the zonae fasciculata and reticularis produce dehydroepiandrosterone.

The base of synthesis of all the adrenal steroid hormones is the cholesterol that is derived from acetyl CoA. After a cytochrome P-450 side chain cleavage enzyme is activated in the mitochondrion, the next conversion is to pregnenolone, while releasing a C6 aldehyde, isocaproaldehyde. The conversion of cholesterol to pregnenolone is the precursor to all the steroidal hormones. Pregnenolone can also be produced from acetate through 24-dehydrocholesterol, but the production is minor.

The pregnenolone can then be converted to progesterone or dehydroepiandrosterone. The production to progesterone, synthesized in the corpus luteum, is accomplished by being acted on by two endoplasmic reticulum enzymes, 3ß-ol dehydrogenase and Δ4,5- isomerase, in the cytosol. In this process, the dehydrogenase acts on the 3-OH group, making a conversion to a 3-keto group. Then the job of the isomerase is to move the double bond from the B ring to the A ring, resulting in progesterone, which has an acetyl group joined at carbon 17 (Devlin, 1992).

In the zona reticularis cells, pregnenolone is acted on by the 17 hydroxylase of the endoplasmic reticulum to create 17ß -hydroxypregnenolone. Then a carbon side chain cleavage system acts upon it by the lyase to create dehydroepiandrosterone, the major adrenal androgen.

Dehydroepiandrosterone (DHEA) is then converted to the C-19 ketosteroid, androstenedione, by an enzyme from the mitochondria of the adrenal cortex, 11 ß-hydroxylase. The androstenedione can then be reduced at the C17 position which results in testosterone, which is the most potent of the adrenal androgens. DHEA can convert to testosterone, bypassing adrostenedione when the DHEA is reduced to its 17-hydroxy derivatives.

Testosterone then can be converted to 17ß-estadiol by being acted upon by the 17-reductase through the aromatase enzyme system. This is accomplished by the by the oxydation of C-19 to 19-hydroxytestosterone. Then the removal of the CH3 at c-10, followed by the aromatization of the A-ring, results in estrone. Estrone and estradiol are interchangeable through a reduction/oxidation which occurs in the liver. Estriol can also be produced when estradiol is acted upon by the 16?-hydroxylase at C-16.

Returning to the conversion of pregnenolone to progesterone, progesterone is a precursor to cortisol (hydrocortisone) and corticosterone. The conversion to corticosterone occurs when hydroxylation at the C21 position occurs to form 11-deoxycorticosterone, followed by a hydroxylation at C11 to produce corticosterone. The corticosterone can then be converted to aldosterone. The conversion to aldosterone, occurring in the adrenal zona glomerulosa cells, requires cytoplasmic 21-hydroxylase, mitochondrial 11ß-hydroxylase and 18-hydroxylase. The 18-alcohol when converted to an aldehyde, results in aldosterone. The conversion to cortisol, occurring in the adrenal z. fasciculata cells requires cytoplasmic 17-hydrolase, 21-hydroxylase, and mitochondrial 11ß-hydroxylase.

It is interesting to note the similarities of the biochemical structure of the precursor derived from the plant sapononin of the Mexican Yam, Dioscorea villosa. With hydrolyzation, these saponins can be converted to sapogenins, such as diosgenin or sarsasapogenin. The same side chain cleavage action mentioned in the conversion of cholesterol to pregnenolone occurs in the diosgenin, resulting in pregnenolone. (Lee, 1993). This natural conversion has great impact on the role of a natural precursor complex. Benefits are addressed in each chapter.

APPENDIX C

WHERE TO GET THE NATURAL PRECURSORS OF DHEA MENTIONED IN THIS BOOK

These products can be ordered from various places, but here are a few suggestions:

I. EMPRISE INTERNATIONAL
   2010 NORTH HIGHWAY 360
   GRAND PRAIRIE, TEXAS 75050
   (214) 641-8829
   (214) 641-8776 Fax

Emprise International has a variety of products derived from Dioscorea.

1) Emprise Plus is a daily supplement, in a proprietary blend, combining extract from Dioscorea with Beta Sitosterol, (which I think is great for lowering cholesterol.

2) Emprise MVP is a proprietary blend of Dioscorea extract with other thermogenic herbs, (which I believe is great for burning fat).

3) Emprise Sport is a Dioscorea extract ideal for those who work out, as it provides a natural anabolic condition.

4) Emprise Firm is a thigh, stomach, arm, and neck cream, combining Dioscorea extract with L-Carnitine and CoEnzyme A to help in the battle of the bulge.

II. PROFESSIONAL AND TECHNICAL SERVICES
    621 SOUTHWEST ALDER, SUITE 900
    PORTLAND, OREGON 97205
    (800) 888-6814
    (205) 226-1010

Professional and Technical Services has two types of products derived from Dioscorea.

1) Pro-Gest cream is a body cream to be applied transdermally.

2) Pro-Gest oil is a sublingual drop to be placed under the tongue.

III. Some pharmacists carry various natural progesterone formulas.

WORKS CITED

Abraham, G.E. "Management of the Premenstrual Tension Syndrome: Rationale for a Nutritional Approach," in Bland, J. 1986: A Year in Nutritional Medicine. New Canaan, CT: Keats Publishing, Inc., 1986.

Aesoph, L.M. "The Five Myths of Aging." Delicious! 10:36-37, 1994.

Amazing Medicines the Drug Companies Don't Want You To Discover! Tempe, Az: University Medical Research Publishers, 1993.

Anderson, D.C., Hopper, B.R., Lasley, B.L. "A Simple Method for the Assay of Eight Steroids in Small Volumes of Plasma." Steroids, 28:179-196, 1976.

Atkins, Dr. "Tired of Aging?" Health Revelations, 1:1-6, 1994.

Arad, Y., Badimon, J.J., Badimon, L. Arteriosclerosis, 9:159, 1989.

Bailey, Covert. Fit or Fat? Boston: Houghton Mifflin Company, 1977.

Barrett-Conner, E., Khaw, K.T., Yen, S.S. "A Prospective Study of DHEA Sulfate, Mortality, and Cardiovascular Disease." New England Journal of Medicine, 315:1519-1524, 1986.

Baulieu, Etienne-Emile, and Kelly, P.A. Hormones:From Molecules to Disease. New York: Hermann Publishers in Arts and Science, 1990.

Bellei, M., Battelli, D., Fornieri, C., Mori, G., Muscatello, U., Lardy, H., and Bobyleva, V. "Changes in Liver Structure and Function After Short-Term and Long-Term Treatment of Rats with Dehydroepiandrosterone." Journal of Nutrition, 122:967-976, 1992.

Berdanier, Carolyn D., John A. Parente, Jr., and Michael K. McIntosh. "Is Dehydroepiandrosterone an antiobesity agent?" FASEB, Vol 7, March 1993.

Berger, S.M. What Your Doctor Didn't Learn in Medical School. New York: Avon Books, 1988.

Better Nutrition for Today's Living. "Health Watch: Staying Thin Helps You Feel Happier, Healthier," April 1994.

Bird, C.E., Masters, V., and Clark, A.F. "Dhea Sulfate: Kinetics of Metabolism in Normal Young men and Women." Clinical Investigative Medicine, 7:119-122, 1984.

Bobyleva, V., Kneer, N. Bellei, M., Battelli, D., Lardy, H. A. "Concerning the Mechanism of Increased Thermogenesis in Rats Treated with Dehydroepiandrosterone." J Bioenerg Biomembr., 25:313-321, 1993.

Bradshaw, John. "Bradshaw On: The Family". Pompano Beach, Florida: Health Communications, Inc., 1988.

Buffington, C.K.., Pourmotabbed, G., Kitabchi, A.E., "Case Report: Amelioration of Insulin Resistance in Diabetes with Dehydroepiandrosterone." Am J. Med. Sci., 306:320-324, 1993.

Bulbrook, R.D., Hayward, J.L., and Spicer, C.C. "Relation Between Urinary Androgen and Corticoid Excretion and Subsequent Breast Cancer." Lancet, 2:395-398, 1971.

Buster, J.E., Casson, P.R. Straughn, A.B., Dale, D., Umstot, E.S., Chiamori, N. and Abraham, G.E. "Postmenopausal Steroid Replacement with Micronized Dehydroepiandrosterone: Preliminary Oral Bioavailability and Does Proportionality Studies." Am J. Obstet Gynecol., 166:1163-1170, 1992.

Cacciari, E., Mazzanti, L., Tasinari, D., Bergamaschi, R., Magnani, C., Zappulla, F., Nanni, G., Cobianchi, C., Ghini, T., Pini, R. "Effects of Sport (Footfall on Growth: Auxological, Anthropometric, and Hormonal Aspects." Eur J. Appl Physiol., 61: 149-158, 1990.

Calabrese, V.P., Isaacs, E.R., Regelson, W. "Dehydroepiandrosterone in Multiple Sclerosis: Positive Effected on the Fatigue Syndrome in a Non-Randomized Study." In The Biologic Role of Dehydroepiandrosterone (DHEA), Kalimi, M. and Regelson, W., Editors. New York: Walter De Gruyter, 1990, pp. 95-100.

Casazza, J.P., Schaffer, W.T., and Veech, R.L. "The Effect of Dehydroepiandrosterone on Liver Metabolites." Journal of Nutrition, 116:304-310, 1986.

Cauley, J.A., Gutai, J.P., Kuller, L.H. Ledonne, D., and Powell, John G. "The Epidemiology of Serum Sex Hormones in Postmenopausal Women." American Journal of Epidemiology, 129:1120-1131.

Cher and Robert Haas, Forever Fit. New York: Bantam Books, 1991.

Chopra, Deepak. Ageless Body, Timeless Mind. New York: Harmony Books, 1993.

Chopra, Deepak. Quantum Healing. New York: Bantam Books, 1989.

Cleary, Margot P. "The Antiobesity Effect of Dehydroepiandrosterone in Rats". Proc Soc Exp Biol Med, 196, #1, 1991: 6-16.

Cleary, M.P., Billheimer, J., Finan, A., Sartin, J.L. and Schwartz, A.G. "Metabolic Consequences of Dehydroepiandrosterone in Lean and Obese Adult Zucker Rats." Horm. Metab. Res., 1984, 16:43-46.

Cleary, M.P. and P.F. Mohan. "Comparison of Dehydroepiandrosterone and Clofibric Acid Treatments in Obese Zucker Rats". Journal of Nutrition. 119:496-501, 1989.

Cleary, M.P., Zabel, T., and Sartin, J.L. "Effects of Short-Term Dehydroepiandrosterone Treatment on Serum and Pancreatic Insulin in Zucker Rats." J. Nutr. 118:382-387, 1988.

Cleary, Margot P. and Joseph F. Zisk. "Anti-Obesity Effect of Two Different Levels of Dehydroepiandrosterone in Lean and Obese Middle-Aged Female Zucker Rats." International Journal of Obesity. 1986, 193-204.

Coleman, D.L. "Dehydroepiandrosterone (DHEA) and Diabetic Syndromes in Mice." In The Biologic Role of Dehydroepiandrosterone (DHEA), Kalimi, M. and Regelson, W., Editors. New York: Walter De Gruyter, 1990, pp. 179-188.

Coleman, D.L., Leiter, E.H. and Applezweig, N. "Therapeutic Effects of Dehydroepiandrosterone Metabolites in Diabetes Mutant Mice (c57BL/KsJ-db/db).*" Endocrinology. 115:239-243, 1984.

Coleman, D.L., Leiter, E.H., Schwizer, R.W. "Therapeutic Effects of Dehydroepiandrosterone (DHEA) in Diabetic Mice." Diabetes. 31:830-833, 1992.

Coleman, D.L., R. W. Schwizer, and E. H. Leiter. "Effect of Genetic Background on the Therapeutic Effects of Dehydroepiandrosterone (DHEA) in Diabetes-Obesity Mutants and in Aged Normal Mice" Diabetes, 33:26-32, 1984.

Consumer Reports on Health. "HDL: 'Good' Cholesterol Looks Even Better." 6:28-30, 1994.

Cooper, K.H. Aerobics. New York: Bantam Books, 1967.

Corpechot, C., Leclerc, P., and Baulieu, E.E., "Neurosteroids: Regulatory Mechanisms in Male Rat Brain During Heterosexual Exposure." Steroids, 45:229-234, 1985.

Corsello, S., "Health Tips Every Woman Should Know." Natural Solutions, Vol. 11, Spring 1994.

Cowan, L.D., et.al. "Breast Cancer Incidence in Women with a History of Progesterone Deficiency." Am.J. Epidemiology, 114:209-217, 1981.

Cutler,W.B. Hysterectomy: Before and After. New York, NY: Harper Perennial, 1988.

Dean, Ward and Morgenthaler, John. Smart Drugs and Nutrients. Santa Cruz, CA: B & J Publications, 1990.

Dean, W., Morgenthaler, J., Fowkes, S.W. Smart Drugs II: The Next Generation. Menlo Park, CA: Health Freedom Publications, 1993.

dePerritti, E. and Forest, M.G. "Pattern of Plasma DHEA Sulfate Levels in Humans from Birth to Adulthood: Evidence for Testicular Production." J. Endocrinology, 57:123-134, 1973.

Devlin, Thomas, M., Editor. Textbook of Biochemistry with Clinical Correlations, Third Edition. New York: Wiley-Liss, 1992.

Diagnostic and Statistics Manual of Mental Disorders. Third Edition, Revised. Washington, DC: American Psychiatric Association, 1987.

Donaldson, K.A. "Health Science News." Total Health. April 1993, 8-9.

Douglas, P.H. and Pinsky, L. The Essential AIDS Fact Book. New York:Pocket Books, 1992.

Dusky, Lorraine. "Progesterone: Safe Antidote for PMS." McCalls Magazine. October 1990, 152-156.

Dyner, T.S., Lang, W., Geaga, J., Golub, A., Stites, D., Wigner, E., Galmarini, M., Masterson, J., and Jacobson, M.A. "An Open-Label Dose-Escalation Trial of Oral Dehydroepiandrosterone Tolerance and Pharmacokinetics in Patients with HIV Disease." Journal of Acquired Immune Deficiency Syndromes, 459-463, 1993.

Eriksson, E., Sunblad, C., Lisjo, P, Modigh, K., and Andersch, B., "Serum Levels of Androgens Are Higher in Women with Premenstrual Irritability and Dysphoria Than in Controls." Psychoneuroendocrinology, 17:195-204, 1992.

Fahraeus, L. Larsson-Cohn U, Wallentin, L. "L-norgestrel and Progesterone Have Different Influences on Plasma Lipoproteins." Eur J. Clin. Invest., 13:447, 1983.

Fassati, P., Fassati, M., Sonka, J. "Dehydroepiandrosterone Sulphate - A New Approach to Some Cases of Angina Pectoris Therapy." Agressologie, 11:445-448, 1970).

Fava, M., Littman, A., and Halperin, P. "Neuroendocrine Correlates of the Type A Behavior Pattern: A Review and new Hypotheses." International J. Psychiatry in Medicine, 17:289-307, 1987.

Fava, M., Rosenbau, J.F., MacLaughlin, R.A., Teasar, G.E., Pollack, M.H., Cohen, L.S., and Hirsch, M. "Dehydroepiandrosterone-Sulfate / Cortisol Ratio in Panic Disorder." Psychiatry Research, 28:345-350, 1989.

Felson, D.T., Zhang, Y., Hannan, M.T., Kile, D.P., Wilson, P.W.F., and Anderson, J.J. "The Effect of Postmenopausal Estrogen Therapy on Bone Density in Elderly Women." The New England Journal of Medicine, 329:1141-1146, 1993.

Feo, F., Pirisi, L., Pascale, R., Daino, L., Frassetto, S., Garcea, R., and Gaspa, L. Cancer Research, 44:3419-3425, 1984.

Feo, F., Pirisi, L., Pascale, R., Daino, L., Franssetto, S., Zanetti, S., and Garcea, R., Toxicol. Pthol., 11:261-268, 1984.

Feo, F., Pirisi, L., Pascale, R., Daino, L., Zanetti, S., LaSpina, V. and Pani, P. In Recent Trends in Chemical Carcinogenesis. Edited by Pani, P., Feo, F., and Columbano, A. E.S.A., Cagliari, pp. 176-196.

Flieger, K. "Why Do We Age?" FDA Consumer. Pp. 20-25, 1988.

Flood, J.F., Smith, G.E., Roberts, E. "Dehydroepiandrosterone and Its Sulfate Enhance Memory Retention in Mice." Brain Research. 447:269-278. 1988.

Fortune, May 1951, p. 87.

Frank, R. T. "The Hormonal Causes of Premenstrual Tension." Arch. Neurol. Psychiatry. 26:1053.

Frenkel, R.A., Slaughter, C.A., Orth, K., Moomaw, C.R., Hicks, S.H., Snuyder, J.M., Bennett, M., Prough, R.A., Putnam, R.S., and Milewich, L. "Peroxisome Proliferation and Induction of Peroxisomal Enzymes in Mouse and Rat Liver by Dehydroepiandrosterone Feeding." J. Steroid Biochem., 35:333-342, 1990.

Glacer, J.L., Brind, J.L., Vogelman, J.H., Eisner, M.J., Dillbeck, M.C., Wallace, R.K., Chopra, D., Orentreich, N. "Elevated Serum Dehydroepiandrosterone Sulfate Levels in Practitioners of the Transcendental Meditation (TM) and TM-Sidhi Programs." Journal of Behavioral Medicine. 15:327-341, 1992.

Gladstar, Rosemary. Herbal Healing for Women. New York: Simon and Schuster, 1993.

Glick, I.D., Quitkin, F.M., and Bennett, S.E. "The Influence of Estrogen, Progestins and Oral Contraceptive on Depression." Gonadal Hormones and Depression, 1990.

Gosnell, Blake A. "Effects of Dietary Dehydroepiandrosterone on FoOd Intake and Body Weight in Rats with Medial Hypothalamic Knife Cuts." Physiology and Behavior. 39:687-691, 1987.

Granholm, N.H., Staber, L.D. and Wilkin, P.J. "Effects of Dehydroepiandrosterone on Obesity and Glucose-6-Phosphate Dehydrogenase Activity in the Lethal Yellow Mouse (Strain 129/Sv - Ay/Aw)" Journal of Experimental Zoology. 242:67-74, 1987.

Granner, Daryl K. "Hormones of the Adrenal Cortex" in Harper's Biochemistry, Murray, R.K., Granner, D.K., Mayes, P.A., Rodwell, V. W. Norwalk, Connecticut: Appleton and Lange, 1988.

Grant, R. "The Mood Cancer." Shape, 38-40, 1994.

Haffner, S.M. Valdez, R. A., Stern, M.P. Katz, M.S. "Obesity, Body Fat Distribution and Sex Hormones in Men." International Journal of Obesity, 17, 643-649, 1993.

Hall, G.M., Perry, L.A., Spector, T.D. "Depressed Levels of Dehydroepiandrosterone Sulphate in Postmenopausal Women with Rheumatoid Arthritis But No Relation with Axial Bone Density." Annals of the Rheumatic Diseases. pp.211-214, 1993.

Hammond, C. B., Jelovsek, F.R., Lee, K.L., Creasman, W.T., Parkman, R.T. "Effects of Long-Term Estrogen Replacement Therapy." Am J. Obstet. Gynecol. 133:525-536, 1979.

Hargrove, J.T., Maxson, W.S., Wentz, A.C., and Burnett, L.S. "Menopausal Hormone Replacement Therapy with Continuous Daily Oral Micronized Estradiol and Progesterone." Obstetrics and Gynecology. 73: 606-612, 1989.

Haug, M., Ouss-Schlegel, M.L., Spetz, J.F., Brain, P.F., Simon, V., Baulieu, E.E., and Robel, P. "Suppressive Effects of Dehydroepiandrosteorne and 3-ß-Methylandrost-5-en-17-one on Attack Towards Lactating Female Intruders by Castrated Male Mice." Physiology and Behavior. 46:955-959, 1989.

Hellerstein, H.K., Hornsten, T.R., Goldbarg, A.G., Burlando, E.H., Friedman, E.H., Hirsch, E.Z., and Marik, S. "The Influence of Active Conditioning upon Subjects with Coronary Artery Disease: Cardiorespiratory Changes during Training in 67 Patients." Canad. Med. Ass. Journal, 96:758-759, 1967.

Helzlsouer, K.J., et.al. "Relationship of Prediagnostic Serum Levels of DHEA." Cancer Research, 52:1-4, 1992.

Hermida, R.C., Halberg, F., and delPorzo, F. "Chronobiologic Pattern Discrimination of Plasma Hormones, Notably DHEA-S and TSH, Classified As Expansive Personality." Chronobiologia. 12:105-136, 1985.

Herrington, D.M., Gordon, G.B., Achuff, S.C., et.al. "Plasma Dehydroepiandrosterone and Dehydroepiandrosterone Sulfate in Patients Undergoing Diagnostic Coronary Angiography." J. Am. Coll. Cardiol, 16:863-870, 1990.

Hopper, B.R. and Yen, S.S. "Circulating Concentrations of DHEA Sulfate During Puberts." J. Clinical Endocrinology and Metabolism, 40:458-461, 1975.

Inoff-Germain, G., Arnold, G.S., Nottelmann, E.D., Susman, E.J., Cutler, G.B., and Chrousos, G.P. "Relations Between Hormone Levels and Observational Measures of Aggressive Behavior in Young Adolescents in Family Interactions." Developmental Psychology. 24:129-139, 1988.

Jacobson, M.A., Fusaro, R.E., Galmarini, M., and Lang, W. "Decreased Serum Dehydroepiandrosterone Is Associated with an Increased Progression of Human Immunodeficiency Virus Infection in Men with CD4 Cell Counts of 200-499." Journal of Infectious Diseases. 164:864-868, 1991.

James, John S. AIDS Treatment News. Berkeley, California: Celestial Arts, 1989.

Janowsky, D.S., Risch, S.C., and Overstreet, D.H. "Psychopharmacologic-Neurotransmitter-Neuroendocrine Interactions in the Study of the Affective Disorders." In Hormones and Depression, Halbreich, U., Ed. New York: Raven Press, 1987.

Kamen, Betty. Hormone Replacement Therapy: Yes or No? Novato California: Nutrition Encounter, Inc., 1993.

Khaw, K.T., Tazuke, S., Barrett-Conner, E. "Cigarette Smoking and Levels of Adrenal Androgens in Post-Menopausal Women. New England Journal of Medicine, 318:1705-1709, 1988.

Klinteberg, B.A., Hallman, J., Oreland, L., Wirsen, A., Levander, S.E., Schalling, D. "Exploring the Connections Between Platelet Monoamine Oxidase Activity and Behavior." Neuropsychobiology. 26:136-145, 1992.

Kurzman, I.D., Macewen, E. G. and Haffa, A.L.M. "Reduction in the Body Weight and Cholesterol in Spontaneously Obese Dogs by Dehydroepiandrosterone." Int. J. Obesity, 14;95-104, 1990.

Langer, Stephen. "Life-Extending Nutrients." Better Nutrition for Today's Living. 1994, pp. 32-37.

Lauersen, N. H. and Stukane, E. Premenstrual Syndrome and You. New York: Simon and Schuster, Inc., 1983.

Leblhuber, F., Neubauer, C., Peichi, M., Reisecker, F., Steinpartz, F.X., Windhager, E., and Dienstl, E. "Age and Sex Differences of Dehydroepiandrosterone Sulfate (DHEAS) and Cortisol (CRT) Plasma Levels in Normal Controls and Alzheimer's Disease." Psychopharmacology. 111:23-26, 1993.

Lee, J.R. "Hormonal and Nutritional Aspects of Osteoporosis." Health and Nutrition. 6:4-8, 1991.

Lee, J.R. "Is Natural Progesterone the Missing Link in Osteoporosis Prevention and Treatment?" Medical Hypotheses. 35:316-318, 1991.

Lee, J.R. Natural Progesterone: The Multiple Roles of a Remarkable Hormone. Sebastopol, California: BLL Publishing, 1993.

Lee, J.R. Optimal Health Guidelines. Sebastopol, California: BLL Publishing, 1993.

Lee, J.R. "Osteoporosis Reversal: The Role of Progesterone." International Clinical Nutrition Review. 10:384-391, 1990.

Lee, J.R. "Significance of Molecular Configuration Specificity: The Case of Progesterone and Osteoporosis." Townsend Letter for Doctors, June 1993, 558-562.

Lee, J.R. "Slowing the Aging Process with Natural Progesterone." Paper in Progress, 1994.

Leighton, B., Tagliaferro, A.R., and Newsholme, E.A. "The Effect of Dehydroepiandrosterone Acetate on Liver Peroxisomal Enzyme Activities of Male and Female Rats." Journal of Nutrition, 117:1287-1290, 1987.

Leiter, E.H., Beamer, W.G., Coleman, D.L., and Longcope, C. "Androgenic and Estrogenic Metabolites in Serum of Mice Fed Dehydroepiandrosterone: Relationship to Antihyperglycemic Effects." Metabolism. 36:863-869, 1987.

Loria, R. M., Regelson, W., Padgett, D.A., "Immune Response Facilitation and Resistance to Virus and Bacterial Infections with Dehydroepiandrosterone (DHEA)." In The Biologic Role of Dehydroepiandrosterone (DHEA), Kalimi, M. and Regelson, W., Editors. New York: Walter De Gruyter, 1990, pp. 107-130.

MacEwen, E., Gregory, and Kurzman, I.D. "Obesity in the Dog: Role of the Adrenal Steroid Dehydroepiandrosterone (DHEA)." J. Nutr. 121:S51-S55, 1991.

MacEwen, E.G., Maki-Haffa, A.L., and Kurzman, I.D. "DHEA Effects on Cholesterol and Lipoproteins." In The Biologic Role of Dehydroepiandrosterone (DHEA), Kalimi, M. and Regelson, W., Editors. New York: Walter De Gruyter, 1990, pp. 299-315.

McIntosh, M.K. and Berdanier, C.D. "Differential Effects of Adrenalectomy and Starvation-Refeeding on Hepatic Lipogenic Responses to Dehydroepiandrosterone and Glucocorticoid in BHE and Sprague-Dawley Rats." J. Nutr. , 118:1011-1017, 1988.

MacIntosh, Anna. "Adrenal Gland Health: A Matter for Menopause." Natural Solutions. 11:5, 1994.

Malinow, M.R. "Effects of Synthetic Glycosides on Cholesterol Absorption." Annals New York Academy of Sciences. 454:23-27, 1985.

"Medical News: Flab-to-Muscle Pill?" American Health, 1988.

Merrill, C.R., Harrington, M.G., Sunderland, T. "Reduced Plasma Dehydroepiandrosterone Concentrations in HIV Infection and Alzheimer's Disease." In The Biologic Role of Dehydroepiandrosterone (DHEA), Kalimi, M. and Regelson, W., Editors. New York: Walter De Gruyter, 1990, pp. 101-105.

Mindell, Earl. Earl Mindell's Herb Bible. New York, NY: Simon and Schuster/Fireside, 1992.

Mirkin, G. "Estrogen in Yams." JAMA, 265:912, 1991.

Mohan, P.F. and Cleary, M.P. "Comparison of Dehydroepiandrosterone and Clofibric Acid Treatments in Obese Zucker Rats." J. Nutr, 119:496-501, 1989.

Mohan, P.F., J.S. Ihnen, B.E. Levin and M.P. Cleary. "Effects of Dehydroepiandrosterone Treatment in Rats with Diet-Induced Obesity." J. Nutr., 1103-1114, 1990.

Moore, M.A., et.al. Carcinogenesis. 7:311-316, 1986.

Morter, M.T. Your Health, Your Choice. Hollywood, Florida: Fell Publishers, Inc., 1993.

Mortola, J.F. and Yen, S.S.C. "The Effects of Oral Dehydroepiandrosterone on Endocrine-Metabolic Parameters in Postmenopausal Women. J. Clin. Endocrinol Metab., 71:696-704, 1990.

Mowrey, Daniel B. The Scientific Validation of Herbal Medicine. New Canaan, Connecticut: Keats Publishing, 1986.

Munk-Jensen, N., Nielsen, S.P., Obel, E.B., Eriksen, P.B. "Reversal of Postmenopausal Vertebral Bone Loss by Oestrogen and Progestagen: A Double Blind Placebo Controlled Study." British Medical Journal, 296:1150-1152.

Murdaugh, C.L., and O'Rourke, R.A. "Coronary Heart Disease in Women: Special Considerations." Curr Probl Cardiol., 13:73-156, 1988).

Nafziger, A.N., Herrington, D.M., and Bush, T.L. "Dehydroepiandrosterone and Dehydroepiandrosterone Sulfate: Their Relation to Cardiovascular Disease." Epidemiologic Reviews, 13:267-293, 1991.

Nafziger, A.N., Jenkins, P.L., Bowlin, S.J. "Dehydroepiandrosterone, Lipids, and Apoproteins Assocations in a Free-Living Population." Circulation, 82:469, 1990.

Nasman, B., Olsson, T., Backstrom, T., Eriksson, S., Grankvist, K., Vitanen, M., and Bucht, G. "Serum Dehydroepiandrosterone Sulfate in Alzheimer's Disease and in Multi-infarct Dementia." Biol. Psychiatry., 30:684-690, 1991.

Nestler, J.E., Barlascini, C. O., Clore, J.N., and Blackard, W.G. "Dehydroepiandrosterone Reduces Serum Low Density Lipoprotein Levels and Body Fat but Does Not Alter Insulin Sensitivity in Normal Men." J. Clin. Endocrinol. & Metab., 66:57-61, 1988.

Nestler, J.E., Clore, J.N., Blackard, W.G. "Dehydroepiandrosterone: the 'Missing Link' Between Hyperinsulinemia and Atherosclerosis?" FASEB J., 6:3073-3075, 1992.

Norton, Terry. "The Menopause Rap Sheet: Symptoms of Menopause." Natural Solutions. 11:4, 1994.

Nottelman, E.D., Susman, E.J., Inoff-Germain, G., Cutler, C.B., Loriaux, D.L., and Chrousos, G.P. "Developmental Processes in Early Adolescence: Relationships Between Adolescent Adjustment Problems and Chronologic Age, Puberty Stage, and Puberty-Related Serum Hormone Levels." J. Pediatrics, pp. 473-480, 1987.

Nowaczynski, W., Fragachan, F., Silah, J., Millette, B., and Genest, J. "Further Evidence of Altered Adrenocortical Function in Hypertension. Dehydroepiandrosterone Excretion Rate." Canadian Journal of Biochemistry, 46:1031-1038, 1968.

Null, Gary. Healing Your Body Naturally. New York: Four Walls, Eight Windows, 1992.

Nyce, J.W., Magee, P.N., and Schwartz, A.G., "Inhibition of 1, Dimethylhydrazine Induced Colon Cancer in Balb/c Mice by Dehydroepiandrosterone." Proc.Am. Assoc Cancer Res., 23:91, 1982.

Nyholt, David. The "Complete" Natural Health Encyclopedia. Alberta Canada: Global Health Pub., 1993.

Orentreich, N., Brind, J.L., and Rizer, R.L. "Age Changes and Sex Differences in Serum Dehydroepiandrosterone Sulfate Concentrations Throughout Adulthood." J. Clin. Endocrinol. Metabl., 59:551-555, 1984.

Osran, H., Reist, C., Cheng-Chung, C., Lifrak, E.T., Chicz-DeMet, A., and Parker, L.N. "Adrenal Androgens and Cortisol in Major Depression." Am Journal of Psychiatry. 150:806-809, 1993.

Parker, L.N., Levin, E.R., Lifrak, E.T. "Evidence for Adrenocortical Adaptation to Severe Illness." Journal of Clinical Endocrinology and Metabolism. 60:947-952, 1985.

Parker, Steve. Eyewitness Science: Human Body. London: Dorling Kindersley, 1993.

Pergola, G.D., Giagulli, V.A., Garruti, G., Cospite, M.R., Giorgino, F., Cignarelli, M. and Giorgino, R. "Low Dehydroepiandrosterone Circulating Levels in Premenopausal Obese Women with Very High Body Mass Index" Metabolism. 40: 187-190, 1991.

Physicians Desk Reference. 48th edition. Montvale, NJ: Medical Economics Data Production Co., 1994.

Pizzorno, L. "Maximize Your Life." Delicious!, 10:30-34, 1994.

Prior, J.C. "Progesterone As a Bone-Trophic Hormone." Endocrine Reviews. 11:386-398, 1990.

Rector-Page, Linda. Healthy Healing: An Alternative Healing Reference. Healthy Healing Publications, 1992.

Regelson, W., Loria, R., and Kalimi, M. "Hormonal Intervention: 'Buffer Hormones' or 'State Dependency'." Annals New York Academy of Sciences. 723:153-160.

Roberts, E. "Dehydroepiandrosterone (DHEA) and Its Sulfate (DHEAS) as Neural Facilitators: Effects on Brain Tissue in Culture and on Memory in Young and Old Mice. A Cyclic GMP Hypothesis of Action of DHEA and DHEAS in Nervous System and Other Tissues." In The Biologic Role of Dehydroepiandrosterone (DHEA), Kalimi, M. and Regelson, W., Editors. New York: Walter De Gruyter, 1990, pp. 13-42.

Roberts, E., Bologa, L., Flood, J.F., and Smith, G.E. "Effects of Dehydroepiandrosterone and Its Sulfate on Brain Tissue in Culture and on

Memory in Mice." Brain Research. 406:357-362. 1987.

Roberts, E. and Fauble, T.J. "Oral Dehydroepiandrosterone in Multiple Sclerosis: Results of a Phase One, Open Study." In The Biologic Role of Dehydroepiandrosterone (DHEA), Kalimi, M. and Regelson, W., Editors. New York: Walter De Gruyter, 1990, pp. 81-93.

Schinazi, R.F., Eriksson, F.H., Arnold, B.H., Leka, P., McGrath, M.S. "Effect of Dehydroepiandrosterone in Lymphocytes and Macrophages Infected with Human Immunodeficiency Viruses." In The Biologic Role of Dehydroepiandrosterone (DHEA), Kalimi, M. and Regelson, W., Editors. New York: Walter De Gruyter, 1990, pp. 157-177.

Schepper, L.D. Human Condition: Critical. Santa Fe, NM:Full of Life Publishing, 1993.

Schwartz, Bob. Diets Still Don't Work!, Houston, Texas: Breatkthru Publishing, 1990.

Simon, Harvey, B. Staying Well: Your Complete Guide to Disease Prevention. Boston: Houghton Mifflin Co., 1992.

Slowinska-Srzednicka, J., Zgliczynski, S., Ciswicka-Sznajderman, M. "Decreased Plasma Dehydroepiandrosterone Sulfate and Dihydrostestosterone Concentrations in Young Men after Myocardial Infarction." Artherosclerosis, 79:197-203, 1989.

Smith, Denny. "Endocrine Complications in HIV Progression." AIDS Treatment News, 140:1-4, 1991.

Smith, Denny. "HIV/Endocrine Update." AIDS Treatment News. 150: 6-8, 1992.

Smith, L.H. "Cholesterol Testing: Is It Worth It?" Total Health. 10-11, 1993.

Smith, M.R., Rudd, B.T., Shirley, A., Rayner, P. H. W., Williams, J. W., Duignan, N.W., and Bertrand, P.V., "A radioimmunoassay for the estimation of serum dehydroepiandrosterone sulfate in normal and pathological serum" , Clin Chim Acta, 65:5 , 1975.

Smith, Trevor. Homeopathic Medicine for Mental Health. Rochester, Vermont: Healing Arts Press, 1989.

Stegmeier, K., Schmidt, F.H., Reinicke, A., and Fahimi, H.D. "Triglyceride Lowering Effect and Induction of Liver Enzymes in Male Rats after

Administation of Hypolipidemic Drugs." Ann. N.Y. Acad. Sci., 386:449-452, 1982.

Steinman, D. "Treating PMS Without Side Effects." Natural Health, 24:52-54, 1994.

Stuart, Mary and Lynnzy Orr, Otherwise Perfect: People and their Problems with Weight. Pompano Beach, Florida: Health Communications, Inc., 1987.

Susman, E.J., Inoff-Germain, G., Nottelmann, E.D., Cutler, G.B., Jr. and Chrousos, G.P. "The Relation of Relative Hormonal Levels and Physical Development and Social-Emotional Behavior in Young Adolescents." Journal of Youth and Adolescence, 14:245-265, 1985.

Tollefson, G.D., Haus, E., Garvey, J.J., Evans, M., and Tusacon, V.G. "Twenty Four Hour Urinary Dehydroepiandrosterone Sulfate in Unipolar Depression Treated with Cognitive and/or Pharmacothrapy." Annals of Clinical Psychiatry. 2:39-45, 1990.

Usiskin, K.S., Butterworth, J. N., Clore, Y.A., Ginsberg, H. N., Blackared, W. G., and Nestler, J. E. "Lack of Effect of Dehydroepiandrosterone in Obese Men." International Journal of Obesity. 14:457-463, 1990.

Wang, D.Y., Bulbrook, R.D., and Clifford, P. "Plasma-Levels of the Sulphate Esters of Dehydroepiandrosterone and Androsterone in Kenyan Men and Their Relation to Cancer of the Nasopharynx." Lancet, 1;1003-1004, 1968.

Wand, D.Y., Bullbrook. R.D., Herian, M., and Hayward, J.L. "Studies on the Sulphate Esters of Measures of Immune Function in Human Immunodeficiency Virus-Related Illness." American Journal of the Medical Sciences. 305:79-83, 1993.

Wright, B.E., Porter, J.R., Browne, E.S. and Svec, F. "Antiglucocorticoid Action of Dehydroepiandrosterone in Young Obese Zucker Rats." International Journal of Obesity. 16:579-583, 1992.

Yamaji, T., Ibayashi, H. "Plasma Dehydroepiandrosterone Sulfate in Normal and Pathological Conditions." J. Clin. Endocrinol., 29:273-278, 1969.

Yang, J.Y., Schwartz, A., Henderson, E.E. "Inhibition of HIV-1 Latency Reactivation by Dehydroepiandrosterone (DHEA) and an Analog of DHEA." AIDS Res Hum Retroviruses. 9:747-754, 1993.

Yen, T.T., Allan, J.A., Pearson, D.V., Acton, J.M., Breenberg, M.M. "Prevention of Obesity in Avy/a Mice by Dehydroepiandrosterone." Lipids, 12:409-413, 1977.

Zagoya, J.C.D. "Studies on the Regulation of Choesterol Metabolism by the Use of the Structural Analogue, Diosgenin." Biolchemical Pharmacology, 20:3473-3480, 1971.

Zumoff, B. "Hormonal Abnormalities in Obesity." Acta Med Scand Suppl. 723:153-160., 1988.

Zumoff, B. and Bradlow, H.L. "Sex Differences in the Metabolism of Dehydroisoandrosterone Sulfate." J. Clin. Endocrinol Metab, 51:334-336, 1980.

Zumoff, B., Levin, J., and Rosenfeld, R.S. "Abnromal 24 Hour Mean Plasma Concentrations of Dehydroepiandrosterone and Dehydroepiandrosterone Sulfate in Women with Primary Operable Breast Cancer." Cancer Res., 41:3360-3363, 1981.

Zumoff, B., Troxler, R.G., O'Connor, J. "Abnormal Hormone Levels in Men with Coronary Artery Disease." Arteriosclerosis, 2:58-67, 1982.

Zwiefel, Jeff. "Art of Successful Weight Management." Total Health, 16:34-36, 1994.

Aching Joints 51
Acidophilus 35
AIDS 135-147
Adrenals   28, 43, 48, 52, 56, 57,
93, 102
Aging 122, 125-127
Alcohol 67, 98, 126
Aldosterone 67
Aloe Vera 140
Alzheimer's Disease 122-134
American Diabetes Association ... 33
Androgens 43, 104,
Anthocyanic Acid 35
Arthritis 19, 92-95
Aspartame 131
Atherosclerosis.... 33, 36, 39, 44, 47
AZT 141
Baby Boomers 123
Bee Pollen 126
Black Cohosh 56,
Butcher's Broom 132
Boron 66
Caffeine 35, 66-67
Calcium 64, 65, 66, 68, 101
Cancer 19, 59, 110, 114-121,
Cardiovascular Disease 48
Chaparral 127
Cholesterol 45, 47, 85-91,
Choline 101
Chromium (GTF) 34-35
CoEnzyme Q 10 132
Coronary Disease 39, 58,
Corticoids 104
Depression 55, 96-107,
DHEA21-28, 38-49, 50-70, 90-91, 92-
95, 102-107, 110-113, 116-117, 123,
129, 132-133, 135-147
DiaBeta 37
Diabetes 19, 32-37
Dioscorea 15, 90

Diosgenin 15, 90
DNA 114-115, 138-139
Dong Quai 56, 126
Dopamine 101
Enoyl-CoA-hydratase 111
Esterone 28, 69
Estradiol 28, 69,
Estrogen51, 54, 58-59, 60, 105, 110,
119
Exercise 63, 101-102, 127
Fat Loss 24
Fat Metabolism 47
Fatigue 39, 137
Fennel 56,
Feverfew........................ 66,
Fluorine 66
Fo-Ti 126
Fountain of Youth 122
Fractures 63
Gallstones 19
Gingko Biloba 126
Ginseng 56
Glucocorticoids 43
Headaches...................... 51,
Heart 38, 123
Heart Disease.................. 19, 33, 40
High Density Lipoproteins 86
Hormonal Changes 28, 54,
Hormonal Imbalances ... 55, 92, 120
Hormone Replacement... 50, 57, 70,
128
Hormones 43, 56, 71-84, 102
Hot Flashes 51, 54,
Hypoglycemia 94, 98
Hypothyroidism 98
Insulin 33-34,
Interferon 140
Kidney Disease 33
L-Arginine 66
L-Lysine 66

Low Density Lipoproteins 86
Libido 51, 68,
Liver 108-113
Magnesium 35, 65, 101
Menopausal Distress 53-54,
Menopause 50-70, 117,
Mexican Yam 15-17, 61, 69, 90, 95,
105
Micronase 37
Mother Hormone 23
Mother Nature 50
MSG 131
Multiple Sclerosis 93-94,
National Cancer Institute
National Cancer Society 115
National Institute of Health 115
Natural Precursor Complex104, 120,
133-134
Niacin 35, 101
Nicotine 43
Norepinephrine 101,
Oatstraw 66
Obesity 18, 21, 47, 117
Oestradiol 28
Oestrogen 68
Osteoporosis 50, 61-70, 92
Ovaries 51, 54
Phenylalanine 101,
Pituitary 54,
PMS 71-84, 102
Pregnancy 119-120
Pregnenolone 69
Progesterone 15, 51, 58-59, 60, 67,
69-70, 102, 105, 119,
Prostate 118
Prozac 104
PSA Test 119
PWA Health Group 143
Selenium 126
Sexual Activity 64-65, 128

Smoking 39, 42, 48, 51, 126
Sodium 54
Sodium Fluoride 66
Steroid 15, 93, 110
Stress 43
Stroke 34, 39, 123
Sugar 66
Testosterone 28, 62, 118
Triglycerides 86-87, 111
Trobriand Islands 16-17
Tumors 59, 121
Type A Behavior 44, 104,
Tyrosine 101
Vanadium 132
Vitamin A 109
Vitamin B 35, 55, 109
Vitamin B1 94
Vitamin B6 .... 94, 101
Vitamin B12 .... 101, 109
Vitamin C35, 55, 66, 68, 89, 101, 140
Vitamin D 55, 66, 68, 86
Vitamin E 89
Vitex 56,
Water Retention 54-55, 59,
Weight Control 19
Weight Loss 18, 24
Yam 16-17,
Yeast 35
Yo Yo Syndrome 20
Zinc 101

ALL INQUIRIES
AND ALL ORDERS
FOR THIS BOOK

BOUNTIFUL HEALTH,
BOUNDLESS ENERGY,
BRILLIANT YOUTH:
THE FACTS ABOUT DHEA

SHOULD BE ADDRESSED TO:

CHARIS PUBLISHING CO., INC.
P. O. BOX 740607
DALLAS, TEXAS 75274
(214) 342-1137

Prices for book :

Single book price	$12.95 each
Two to 20 copies	9.95 each
Over 20 copies	7.95 each

Please send _____copies @ $_____
Texas residents add 8.25% tax _____
Shipping/Handling   _____
        $2.25 per book
        $.50 per book for 2-20
        No charge for ove 20 books
TOTAL ENCLOSED $_____

SHIPPING ADDRESS:

NAME _____

ADDRESS _____

CITY, STATE, ZIP _____

PHONE NUMBER _____